GROWING MEDICINAL HERBS FOR BEGINNERS

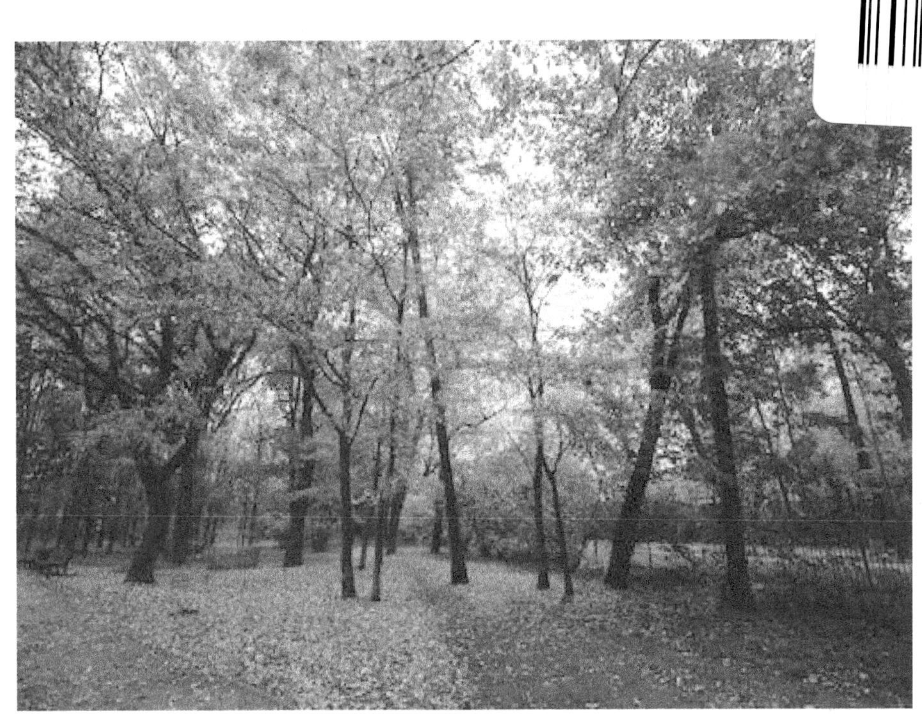

DR. VICKIE STOCK

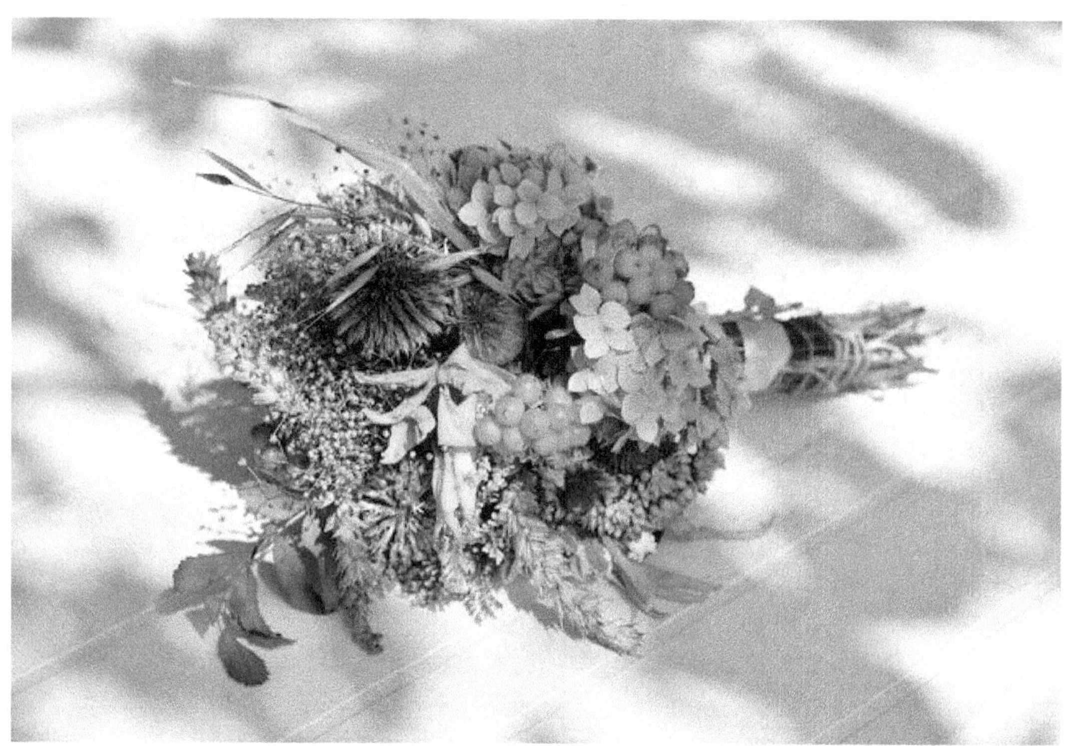

TABLE OF CONTENT

CHAPTER ONE: Introduction to Medicinal Herbs

Understanding Medicinal Herbs

Medicinal herbs, also known as medicinal plants or healing herbs, have been an integral part of human history for thousands of years. These plants, endowed with therapeutic properties, have played a crucial role in traditional medicine systems across cultures and continue to captivate the interest of modern herbalists and health enthusiasts. Understanding medicinal herbs involves delving into their diverse qualities, historical significance, and the various ways they contribute to health and wellness.

Medicinal herbs can be defined as plants that possess pharmacological compounds with the potential to alleviate or prevent ailments in the human body. These plants are a rich source of bioactive compounds, such as alkaloids, flavonoids, and essential oils, which exhibit medicinal properties. The use of medicinal herbs dates back to ancient civilizations, where knowledge about their healing properties was passed down through generations.

The historical significance of medicinal herbs is profound, with each culture contributing to a vast repository of herbal knowledge. In ancient China, traditional Chinese medicine embraced herbs like ginseng and licorice for their adaptogenic and anti-inflammatory properties.

Ayurveda, the traditional medicine system of India, relied heavily on herbs such as turmeric, neem, and ashwagandha for their healing capabilities. Similarly, indigenous cultures worldwide cultivated a deep understanding of their local flora, utilizing plants like echinacea, yarrow, and elderberry for various medicinal purposes.

The benefits of medicinal herbs are multifaceted, encompassing physical, mental, and even spiritual well-being. Many herbs exhibit antioxidant properties, helping the body combat oxidative stress and reduce the risk of chronic diseases.

For instance, herbs like rosemary and oregano are rich in antioxidants that may contribute to overall health. Moreover, certain herbs possess anti-inflammatory effects, offering a natural alternative to pharmaceutical solutions for conditions like arthritis and inflammatory disorders. The sustainable aspect of growing and utilizing medicinal herbs is another key benefit.

Unlike synthetic pharmaceuticals, which often have environmental impacts, herbs can be grown organically, fostering a more sustainable approach to healthcare. Cultivating medicinal herbs in home gardens or on small farms empowers individuals to take charge of their health in an eco-friendly manner.

Understanding medicinal herbs also involves recognizing the holistic nature of herbal medicine. Rather than merely targeting specific symptoms, herbal remedies often address the root causes of imbalances within the body. This holistic approach aligns with the concept of wellness and emphasizes the interconnectedness of various bodily systems.

To embark on the journey of understanding medicinal herbs, one must explore their diverse uses and applications. From culinary herbs like basil and thyme, which add flavor to dishes while offering health benefits, to more potent medicinal plants like echinacea and chamomile, each herb has a unique profile of active compounds.

Exploring the world of medicinal herbs also requires an understanding of plant chemistry. The active constituents in herbs interact with the body in intricate ways, influencing physiological processes and promoting health. This knowledge forms the basis for creating herbal preparations such as teas, tinctures, and salves, each tailored to harness the healing potential of specific herbs.

Understanding medicinal herbs is a journey that encompasses history, culture, science, and a profound appreciation for the healing power of nature. As individuals increasingly seek natural and sustainable approaches to healthcare, medicinal herbs emerge as a valuable resource for promoting well-being. Whether incorporated into daily cuisine or used to formulate therapeutic remedies, medicinal herbs invite us to reconnect with the ancient wisdom that recognizes nature as a healer and source of vitality.

Definition and Importance of Medicinal Herbs

Medicinal herbs, often referred to as healing herbs or medicinal plants, constitute a diverse array of plant species that possess therapeutic properties. These plants have been integral to various traditional medicine systems across the globe, serving as the foundation for natural healing practices.

The definition of medicinal herbs lies in their ability to produce bioactive compounds with potential medicinal benefits, contributing to the well-being of humans in profound ways. At its core, the term "medicinal herbs" encompasses a broad spectrum of plant life that holds therapeutic value. These plants produce a myriad of chemical compounds, such as alkaloids, flavonoids, terpenes, and essential oils, each carrying distinct healing properties.

From the soothing effects of chamomile to the immune-boosting qualities of echinacea, medicinal herbs showcase a remarkable diversity in their chemical composition and applications.

The importance of medicinal herbs is deeply rooted in their historical and cultural significance. Throughout the annals of human civilization, communities around the world have recognized the healing potential of plants and integrated them into their traditional healing practices.

Ancient Chinese medicine, Ayurveda in India, Native American herbalism, and European herbal traditions are just a few examples of how medicinal herbs have played pivotal roles in diverse cultures. The importance of medicinal herbs extends beyond historical contexts to the contemporary era, where there is a growing awareness and interest in natural and holistic approaches to health.

In an age marked by synthetic pharmaceuticals, medicinal herbs offer a compelling alternative, often with fewer side effects and a more harmonious interaction with the body. This shift towards herbal remedies aligns with a desire for sustainable, plant-based solutions that promote wellness without causing harm to the environment or the body.

One of the primary advantages of medicinal herbs lies in their holistic nature. Rather than isolating and targeting specific symptoms, medicinal herbs often address the underlying causes of imbalances within the body.

This holistic approach resonates with the broader concept of wellness, acknowledging the interconnectedness of physical, mental, and emotional aspects of health. It promotes a more comprehensive understanding of the body's intricate systems and encourages practices that support overall well-being.

The cultivation and use of medicinal herbs contribute significantly to sustainable living practices. Unlike pharmaceuticals, which can have ecological repercussions, medicinal herbs can be grown organically, reducing the environmental impact of healthcare practices.

Home gardens, community herb plots, and small-scale herb farms empower individuals to take control of their health in an eco-friendly manner, fostering a deeper connection to the natural world. The importance of medicinal herbs also extends to their economic value. The herbal industry, including the production of herbal supplements, teas, essential oils, and other herbal products, has witnessed substantial growth.

This not only provides economic opportunities for farmers and businesses but also contributes to a diversified and resilient healthcare system.

The definition and importance of medicinal herbs intertwine with the rich tapestry of human history, cultural practices, and the evolving landscape of healthcare. These plants offer a holistic approach to healing, addressing not just symptoms but the root causes of health imbalances.

As society increasingly values sustainability and seeks alternatives to conventional medicine, medicinal herbs emerge as a valuable resource, inviting individuals to embrace the inherent healing properties of nature for a healthier and more balanced life.

Historical Significance of Medicinal Herbs

The historical significance of medicinal herbs is a captivating journey through the annals of human civilization, weaving a tapestry of ancient wisdom, cultural practices, and the profound relationship between humanity and the healing power of nature. From the earliest civilizations to the present day, medicinal herbs have played a pivotal role in shaping healthcare practices and influencing cultural traditions.

The roots of the historical significance of medicinal herbs stretch back to ancient times when humans first discovered the therapeutic properties of plants through trial and error. The use of medicinal herbs is deeply embedded in the traditions of various cultures, each contributing to a vast repository of herbal knowledge.

In ancient China, herbal medicine was an integral component of traditional Chinese medicine (TCM), with herbs like ginseng, astragalus, and licorice being revered for their adaptogenic and immune-boosting properties. Similarly, Ayurveda, the traditional medicine system of India, relied heavily on herbs such as turmeric, neem, and ashwagandha to restore balance to the body and mind.

In ancient Egypt, medicinal herbs were documented in the Ebers Papyrus, one of the oldest known medical texts dating back to around 1550 BCE. Herbs like aloe vera and garlic were recognized for their healing properties, showcasing the ancient Egyptians' understanding of herbal medicine.

The Greeks, with prominent figures like Hippocrates, emphasized the importance of herbs in medicine. Hippocrates, often regarded as the father of Western medicine, famously stated, "Let food be thy medicine, and medicine be thy food," underscoring the significance of natural remedies, including medicinal herbs.

During the Middle Ages, the knowledge of medicinal herbs was preserved and expanded upon by Islamic scholars. The works of figures like Avicenna, a Persian polymath, played a crucial role in advancing herbal medicine.

Herbals, illustrated manuscripts detailing the properties and uses of medicinal plants, became popular during this period, with the "Herbarium" of Apuleius Platonicus being one such notable example. In the Americas, indigenous cultures developed a profound understanding of their local flora, utilizing medicinal herbs for healing purposes.

Native American herbalism incorporated plants like echinacea, goldenseal, and sage into their medicinal repertoire. The knowledge of herbal remedies was passed down through oral traditions, highlighting the intimate connection between nature and healing in indigenous cultures.

The Renaissance period saw a resurgence of interest in herbalism, with herbal gardens cultivated for both medicinal and aesthetic purposes. Herbalists like John Gerard and Nicholas Culpeper made significant contributions, compiling herbal texts that served as references for generations to come. Culpeper's "Complete Herbal," published in the 17th century, remains a classic in herbal literature.

The historical significance of medicinal herbs continued to evolve with the exploration and exchange of plants during the Age of Discovery. Plants like cinchona, the source of quinine for treating malaria, and various medicinal herbs from the New World were introduced to Europe, influencing medical practices globally.

In the modern era, the rediscovery of herbal medicine gained momentum, driven by a growing interest in natural and holistic approaches to health. Scientific advancements have allowed researchers to explore and validate the therapeutic properties of medicinal herbs, bridging the gap between traditional knowledge and evidence-based medicine.

The historical significance of medicinal herbs is not confined to the past; it resonates in the present as societies rediscover the value of natural remedies. The enduring legacy of herbal traditions serves as a reminder of the profound connection between humans and the plant kingdom, offering a timeless source of healing and well-being.

As individuals today seek alternatives to synthetic pharmaceuticals, the historical wisdom embedded in medicinal herbs continues to shape the landscape of healthcare, fostering a harmonious relationship between humanity and the healing bounty of nature.

Benefits of Growing Medicinal Herbs

The decision to cultivate medicinal herbs goes beyond the realms of gardening; it is a holistic embrace of nature's pharmacy and a journey towards sustainable health and wellness. Growing medicinal herbs offers a multitude of benefits that extend from the garden to the kitchen and, ultimately, to the well-being of individuals and communities. Here, we explore the diverse advantages that come with cultivating these herbal treasures.

Health and Wellness:

Cultivating medicinal herbs provides a direct and accessible source of natural remedies for various health concerns. Herbs like lavender, chamomile, and lemon balm offer relaxation and stress relief, while others such as echinacea and elderberry contribute to immune system support. The therapeutic properties of these plants can be harnessed through teas, tinctures, and salves, promoting a natural and preventive approach to health.

Sustainable Living:

Medicinal herb cultivation aligns with sustainable living practices. Herbs are often resilient, requiring fewer synthetic inputs like pesticides and fertilizers. Embracing organic and permaculture principles in herb gardening not only reduces the environmental impact but also fosters a harmonious coexistence with the ecosystem. This sustainable approach is in stark contrast to the resource-intensive processes involved in pharmaceutical production.

Economic Considerations:

Growing medicinal herbs presents economic opportunities for individuals and communities. The herbal products industry, encompassing supplements, essential oils, and herbal teas, continues to witness growth. Small-scale herb farms and local herbalists can contribute to the local economy while providing consumers with high-quality, locally sourced products. The economic benefits extend beyond mere cultivation to processing, packaging, and marketing of herbal goods.

Culinary Delights:

Many medicinal herbs double as flavorful additions to culinary creations. Herbs like basil, thyme, and rosemary not only bring aromatic richness to dishes but also offer nutritional value.

Integrating medicinal herbs into daily cuisine is a delightful way to enhance flavor while reaping the health benefits. This dual-purpose aspect of medicinal herbs adds a practical and enjoyable dimension to their cultivation.

Biodiversity and Ecosystem Support:

Medicinal herb gardens contribute to biodiversity by attracting beneficial insects and pollinators. Bees, butterflies, and other pollinators play a crucial role in maintaining ecosystem health and supporting food production. Creating a habitat that welcomes these creatures enhances the overall resilience of the garden and its surrounding environment.

Educational Opportunities:

Cultivating medicinal herbs provides a rich learning experience for individuals and communities. It encourages the exploration of herbal traditions, plant identification, and the art of herbal preparations. Educational initiatives around herbalism and botany can empower people with knowledge about the local flora and its potential applications, fostering a deeper connection to nature.

Empowerment and Self-Sufficiency:

Growing medicinal herbs empowers individuals to take charge of their health and well-being. The ability to cultivate, harvest, and prepare herbal remedies instills a sense of self-sufficiency. This empowerment is particularly valuable in times when individuals seek alternatives to mainstream healthcare or wish to complement conventional treatments with natural remedies.

Aesthetic Beauty:

Medicinal herb gardens are not only functional but also visually appealing. Many herbs, with their diverse foliage, colors, and fragrances, contribute to the aesthetic charm of a garden. Creating a space that is both therapeutic and beautiful enhances the overall experience of gardening and encourages spending time outdoors.

The benefits of growing medicinal herbs extend far beyond the physical act of gardening. They encompass health, sustainability, economic opportunities, and a profound connection to nature. Whether one has a small herb garden on a balcony or a larger plot of land, cultivating medicinal herbs offers a holistic approach to living that integrates the principles of well-being, environmental stewardship, and a harmonious relationship with the natural world.

Choosing the Right Location for Sustainable Living

Selecting the appropriate location is a pivotal step in the journey towards sustainable living, as it significantly influences the environmental impact, quality of life, and overall success of sustainable practices. Whether establishing a new residence, a community project, or a business, the geographic setting plays a crucial role in determining the feasibility and effectiveness of sustainability initiatives. This exploration delves into the key factors to consider when choosing the right location for sustainable living.

Climate and Bioregion:

The climate and bioregion of a location are fundamental considerations in sustainable living. Understanding the local climate influences decisions related to energy-efficient home design, appropriate landscaping practices, and the selection of native plants that thrive in the region.

Additionally, embracing the principles of bioregionalism entails aligning human activities with the natural ecosystems of the area, promoting a more sustainable and resilient relationship with the environment.

Renewable Energy Potential:

Assessing the renewable energy potential of a location is paramount for sustainable living. Areas with abundant sunlight may be ideal for solar energy, while regions with consistent wind patterns may be suitable for wind power.

Analyzing the renewable energy resources available enables individuals and communities to make informed decisions about incorporating solar panels, wind turbines, or other sustainable energy systems into their living or working spaces.

Water Availability and Management:

Water is a precious resource, and its availability and management are critical aspects of sustainable living. Choosing a location with a sustainable water supply ensures resilience in the face of changing climate patterns.

Implementing water-efficient practices, rainwater harvesting, and eco-friendly landscaping contribute to responsible water management. Understanding the local watershed and water conservation measures is essential for minimizing environmental impact.

Proximity to Resources and Local Services:

The proximity to essential resources and local services is a practical consideration for sustainable living. Choosing a location close to farmers' markets, local produce, and community-supported agriculture facilitates access to fresh, locally sourced food. Additionally, being near public transportation, schools, and healthcare services reduces the environmental impact associated with commuting and promotes community engagement.

Biodiversity and Conservation Values:

A location's biodiversity and conservation values contribute to its ecological sustainability. Areas rich in biodiversity often have unique ecosystems that require protection. Choosing a location with a commitment to conservation supports efforts to preserve natural habitats, protect endangered species, and maintain ecological balance. Living in harmony with local flora and fauna enhances the overall ecological health of the chosen location.

Land Use and Zoning Regulations:

Understanding land use and zoning regulations is essential for navigating sustainable living initiatives. Some areas may have zoning regulations that restrict certain sustainable practices, such as rainwater harvesting or the installation of renewable energy systems. Familiarity with local regulations ensures compliance and may also provide opportunities to advocate for sustainable practices within the community.

Community and Social Dynamics:

The community and social dynamics of a location influence the success of sustainable living initiatives. Choosing a location with like-minded individuals who share a commitment to sustainability fosters a supportive community. Engaging with local community organizations, participating in sustainability initiatives, and collaborating with neighbors contribute to a sense of belonging and shared values.

Natural Hazards and Resilience:

Assessing the susceptibility to natural hazards is crucial for building resilience in sustainable living. Understanding the risks associated with earthquakes, floods, wildfires, or other environmental challenges allows individuals and communities to implement strategies for disaster preparedness and sustainable rebuilding. Incorporating resilience measures into the planning process ensures that sustainable practices persist in the face of unforeseen events.

Sunlight Requirements

Understanding sunlight requirements is paramount when embarking on sustainable living, especially in the context of gardening, agriculture, and energy production. Sunlight, with its abundance and renewability, serves as a foundational resource for life on Earth. This exploration delves into the significance of sunlight requirements in various aspects of sustainable living, emphasizing its role in fostering growth, energy production, and overall well-being.

Plant Growth and Agriculture:

Sunlight is a crucial determinant of successful plant growth and agricultural productivity. Plants undergo photosynthesis, a process that converts sunlight into energy, enabling them to produce their own food. Different plants have varying sunlight requirements, categorized into full sun, partial sun, or shade. Understanding these requirements is essential for planning sustainable gardens and agricultural practices. Optimal sunlight exposure not only supports plant health but also influences factors like flowering, fruiting, and overall yield.

Solar Energy Harvesting:

Sustainable energy production is closely tied to harnessing the power of sunlight. Solar panels, or photovoltaic cells, capture sunlight and convert it into electricity. The efficiency of solar energy systems is directly influenced by the amount and duration of sunlight received.

When choosing a location for solar installations, factors such as the angle of sunlight exposure, potential shading, and regional solar irradiance play critical roles. Strategically positioning solar panels to maximize sunlight absorption enhances the effectiveness of solar energy harvesting.

Passive Solar Design in Architecture:

Sunlight plays a pivotal role in passive solar design, an architectural approach that utilizes natural sunlight for heating, cooling, and lighting buildings. Proper orientation of windows, incorporation of thermal mass, and the use of shading devices are integral elements of passive solar design. By leveraging sunlight for heating during winter and implementing shading strategies to minimize heat gain in summer, passive solar design contributes to energy efficiency, reducing the reliance on artificial heating and cooling systems.

Circadian Rhythms and Human Well-Being:

Sunlight exposure is crucial for maintaining healthy circadian rhythms, the internal biological clocks that regulate sleep-wake cycles and various physiological processes in humans. Exposure to natural sunlight, especially in the morning, helps synchronize circadian rhythms, promoting better sleep quality and overall well-being. Incorporating daylight into indoor spaces through thoughtful architectural design enhances human comfort and productivity while minimizing the need for artificial lighting during daylight hours.

Sustainable Gardening Practices:

Sustainable gardening practices emphasize working in harmony with natural elements, and sunlight is a primary consideration. Choosing appropriate plant varieties based on their sunlight requirements, implementing companion planting strategies to optimize sunlight exposure, and utilizing organic soil amendments contribute to sustainable gardening. Additionally, incorporating rainwater harvesting and mulching practices helps retain soil moisture, creating a more resilient and water-efficient garden.

Seasonal Considerations:

Sunlight availability varies with the seasons, influencing sustainable practices throughout the year. Understanding the changing angles of the sun during different seasons is crucial for optimizing sunlight exposure. This knowledge informs decisions on planting schedules, solar panel tilt angles, and passive solar design strategies. Adapting sustainable practices to seasonal sunlight variations ensures that resources are utilized efficiently and effectively.

Sustainable Forest Management:

Sunlight plays a critical role in sustainable forest management. Forest ecosystems depend on sunlight for photosynthesis, supporting the growth of trees and the myriad plant and animal species within. Sustainable logging practices consider sunlight requirements for regeneration, promoting selective logging and reforestation strategies that maintain the ecological balance. Preserving natural sunlight access in forested areas contributes to biodiversity conservation and overall ecosystem health.

Educational and Recreational Spaces:

Sunlight is a key consideration in the design of educational and recreational spaces. Incorporating natural daylight into learning environments enhances the overall well-being and cognitive performance of students. Similarly, ensuring sunlight access in recreational areas, such as parks and outdoor sports facilities, promotes physical activity, mental health, and community engagement.

Soil Quality and Drainage:

The health of the soil is a critical determinant of success in various sustainable living practices, including gardening, agriculture, and ecosystem restoration. Soil quality encompasses a range of physical, chemical, and biological attributes that influence its ability to support plant growth, water retention, and nutrient cycling.

Drainage, on the other hand, is a crucial aspect that determines how effectively water moves through the soil, preventing waterlogging and supporting aeration. This exploration delves into the significance of soil quality and drainage in sustainable living, emphasizing their roles as the foundation for robust and resilient ecosystems.

Nutrient Availability and Plant Health:

Soil quality directly impacts nutrient availability to plants, influencing their health and productivity. Healthy soil teems with microorganisms that break down organic matter, releasing essential nutrients for plant uptake.

Sustainable living practices involve maintaining and enhancing soil fertility through the addition of organic amendments, cover cropping, and crop rotation. By ensuring a balance of nutrients, soil quality supports thriving plant life without the need for excessive synthetic fertilizers.

Water Retention and Conservation:

The ability of soil to retain water is a key factor in sustainable living, particularly in regions prone to water scarcity. Soil quality plays a pivotal role in water retention by influencing its texture, structure, and organic content. Well-structured soil with good organic matter content retains moisture efficiently, reducing the need for excessive irrigation. Sustainable water management practices, such as mulching and rainwater harvesting, further contribute to water conservation and soil health.

Erosion Control and Soil Stability:

Sustainable living practices prioritize erosion control and soil stability to prevent the loss of valuable topsoil.

Healthy vegetation, cover cropping, and contour plowing are strategies that enhance soil structure and reduce erosion. Additionally, incorporating perennial plants with deep root systems helps bind the soil, preventing it from being washed away during heavy rains. By safeguarding against soil erosion, sustainable practices maintain the integrity of the land and promote long-term environmental health.

Microbial Diversity and Soil Biology:

The health of the soil is intricately tied to its microbial diversity and overall biological activity. Sustainable living practices recognize the importance of fostering a thriving soil ecosystem, encompassing bacteria, fungi, and other microorganisms. These soil inhabitants contribute to nutrient cycling, disease suppression, and the formation of symbiotic relationships with plant roots. Practices such as avoiding excessive tillage and incorporating organic matter support a diverse and resilient soil biology.

Drainage and Aeration:

Proper drainage is essential for sustainable living, as it prevents waterlogging and ensures adequate oxygen supply to plant roots. Soil compaction, often a result of heavy machinery or excessive foot traffic, can impede drainage and lead to a decrease in soil aeration. Sustainable gardening and agricultural practices emphasize minimizing soil disturbance, utilizing cover crops, and incorporating organic matter to enhance soil structure and promote optimal drainage.

Regenerative Agriculture Practices:

Regenerative agriculture represents a holistic approach to farming that prioritizes soil health and regeneration. Cover cropping, rotational grazing, and agroforestry are regenerative practices that enhance soil quality, improve water retention, and support biodiversity. By mimicking natural ecosystems, regenerative agriculture fosters resilient and sustainable food production systems that prioritize the long-term health of the soil and the surrounding environment.

Contaminant Avoidance and Remediation:

Sustainable living practices involve avoiding the use of harmful chemicals and pollutants that can degrade soil quality. Organic farming, for example, eschews synthetic pesticides and fertilizers in favor of natural alternatives. In cases where soil contamination has occurred, sustainable remediation techniques, such as phytoremediation using specific plant species, can be employed to mitigate the impact and restore soil health.

Permaculture Principles:

Permaculture, a design system that integrates ecological principles into human habitats, places a strong emphasis on soil health and water management. Permaculture practices include creating swales for water retention, implementing food forests to enhance biodiversity, and utilizing companion planting to optimize nutrient cycling. By applying permaculture principles, individuals can design sustainable living spaces that function as self-sustaining ecosystems.

Selecting Suitable Herbs:

Choosing the right herbs is a foundational step in establishing a successful and rewarding herbal garden. Whether you're a seasoned gardener or a beginner embarking on the journey of cultivating medicinal and culinary herbs, the selection process is crucial to ensure optimal growth, yield, and utilization of these versatile plants. This exploration delves into the considerations for selecting suitable herbs, considering factors such as climate, soil conditions, and intended uses.

Climate and Growing Conditions:

The first and foremost consideration in selecting herbs is the local climate and growing conditions. Herbs, like all plants, have specific temperature, sunlight, and moisture requirements. Some herbs thrive in full sun, while others prefer partial shade.

Understanding the climate zone and microclimates of your region helps in choosing herbs that are well-suited to the environmental conditions. For example, Mediterranean herbs such as rosemary and thyme thrive in sunny, well-drained environments, while mint and parsley may prefer slightly shaded and moister conditions.

Soil Quality and pH:

Different herbs have varying soil preferences, and understanding the soil quality and pH of your garden is essential. Herbs generally prefer well-draining soil with good aeration. Testing the soil's pH helps determine whether it is acidic, neutral, or alkaline, allowing you to select herbs that are adapted to those conditions. For instance, lavender and sage prefer alkaline soils, while herbs like cilantro and chives thrive in neutral to slightly acidic conditions.

Intended Use and Culinary Preferences:

Consider the intended use of the herbs in your garden, whether it's for culinary purposes, medicinal applications, or aromatic qualities. Culinary herbs like basil, oregano, and thyme add flavor and depth to dishes, while medicinal herbs such as chamomile and echinacea have specific health benefits. Planning your herb garden based on these intended uses ensures that you cultivate a diverse and purposeful selection of herbs tailored to your needs.

Space and Container Gardening:

The available space and your gardening setup influence the selection of herbs. If you have limited space, herbs like mint and chives are well-suited for container gardening, providing flexibility in placement and managing their potentially invasive growth. Consider the growth habits of the herbs, such as the spreading nature of mint or the vertical growth of rosemary, to optimize space utilization and create an aesthetically pleasing garden layout.

Companion Planting and Pest Management:

Harnessing the principles of companion planting can enhance the health and resilience of your herb garden. Certain herbs, when planted together, can deter pests or enhance each other's growth. For example, planting basil alongside tomatoes can improve the flavor of the tomatoes and deter pests that affect both plants. Understanding these beneficial interactions contributes to the overall sustainability of your garden.

Perennial vs. Annual Herbs:

Consider the life cycle of the herbs you choose, distinguishing between perennial and annual varieties. Perennial herbs like sage and thyme persist through multiple growing seasons, providing long-term yields.

Annual herbs, such as basil and cilantro, complete their life cycle within a single growing season. Integrating a mix of perennial and annual herbs ensures a continuous harvest and dynamic garden composition.

Aromatic Qualities and Ornamental Appeal:

Many herbs are prized for their aromatic qualities and ornamental appeal. Herbs like lavender, rosemary, and mint release delightful fragrances when touched or brushed against, contributing to sensory enjoyment in the garden. Additionally, herbs with attractive foliage, flowers, or unique growth habits can enhance the visual appeal of your garden, making it a welcoming and aesthetically pleasing space.

Cultural and Historical Significance:

Exploring the cultural and historical significance of herbs adds depth and meaning to your garden. Herbs have been used for centuries in various cultures for culinary, medicinal, and spiritual purposes. Understanding the traditional uses of herbs can inspire a connection to heritage and contribute to a diverse and culturally rich herb garden.

Common Medicinal Herbs for Beginners:

Embarking on the journey of cultivating medicinal herbs offers a gateway to the world of natural remedies and holistic well-being. For beginners, selecting common medicinal herbs with versatile uses and straightforward cultivation requirements is an excellent starting point. These herbs not only provide health benefits but also serve as a foundation for exploring the rich traditions of herbalism. This exploration delves into a selection of common medicinal herbs for beginners, highlighting their uses, growing conditions, and simple preparations.

Peppermint (Mentha x piperita):

- ➢ Uses: Peppermint is prized for its soothing properties, aiding digestion and relieving symptoms of indigestion. It also has antimicrobial and anti-inflammatory properties.
- ➢ Growing Conditions: Peppermint thrives in well-drained soil and partial shade. It is known for its vigorous growth, making it suitable for container gardening to prevent spreading.
- ➢ Preparation: Peppermint tea is a popular and easy preparation. Simply steep fresh or dried leaves in hot water for a refreshing and digestive-friendly beverage.

Lavender (Lavandula spp.):

- ➢ Uses: Lavender is renowned for its calming and aromatic qualities. It is commonly used in aromatherapy, and its flowers can be infused into various preparations for relaxation.
- ➢ Growing Conditions: Lavender prefers well-drained soil and full sunlight. It is a hardy perennial that adds ornamental value to gardens.
- ➢ Preparation: Lavender-infused oil or tea is simple to make and can be used for aromatherapy, as a skin-soothing agent, or added to baths for a calming experience.

Chamomile (Matricaria chamomilla):

- ➢ Uses: Chamomile is celebrated for its calming and sleep-inducing properties. It also has anti-inflammatory and digestive benefits.
- ➢ Growing Conditions: Chamomile prefers well-drained soil and full sunlight. It is an annual herb with daisy-like flowers.
- ➢ Preparation: Chamomile tea is a classic preparation. Drying the flowers and steeping them in hot water creates a mild and soothing infusion.

Echinacea (Echinacea purpurea):

- ➢ Uses: Echinacea is valued for its immune-boosting properties. It is often used to support the body during colds and flu.
- ➢ Growing Conditions: Echinacea thrives in well-drained soil and full to partial sunlight. It is a hardy perennial with distinctive purple flowers.
- ➢ Preparation: Echinacea tinctures or teas are common preparations. The roots, flowers, or leaves can be utilized for immune system support.

Rosemary (Rosmarinus officinalis):

- ➢ Uses: Rosemary is known for its cognitive and memory-enhancing properties. It also has antioxidant and anti-inflammatory benefits.
- ➢ Growing Conditions: Rosemary prefers well-drained soil and full sunlight. It is a perennial herb with needle-like leaves.
- ➢ Preparation: Infusing rosemary in oil for culinary use or as a massage oil is a simple method. Rosemary tea can also be made by steeping fresh or dried leaves.

Calendula (Calendula officinalis):

- ➢ Uses: Calendula is valued for its skin-soothing and anti-inflammatory properties. It is often used in salves, creams, and ointments.
- ➢ Growing Conditions: Calendula thrives in well-drained soil and full to partial sunlight. It is an annual herb with vibrant orange or yellow flowers.
- ➢ Preparation: Calendula-infused oil is a versatile preparation. The oil can be used topically for skin conditions or incorporated into homemade skincare products.

Lemon Balm (Melissa officinalis):

Uses: Lemon balm is known for its calming and mood-lifting effects. It also has antiviral and digestive benefits.

Growing Conditions: Lemon balm prefers well-drained soil and partial shade. It is a hardy perennial with lemon-scented leaves.

Preparation: Lemon balm tea is a delightful and easy preparation. Drying the leaves and steeping them in hot water creates a fragrant and soothing infusion.

Thyme (Thymus vulgaris):

- Uses: Thyme is recognized for its antimicrobial properties and is often used for respiratory health. It also has antioxidant and culinary uses.
- Growing Conditions: Thyme prefers well-drained soil and full sunlight. It is a perennial herb with small, aromatic leaves.
- Preparation: Thyme-infused honey or thyme tea can be made by steeping fresh or dried leaves. This preparation is commonly used for respiratory support.

These common medicinal herbs offer a well-rounded introduction to the world of herbalism for beginners. They are versatile, easy to grow, and provide a foundation for exploring herbal preparations and applications. Whether used for teas, infused oils, or topical applications, these herbs bring the benefits of nature's pharmacy to your garden and home. As you delve into cultivating and using these medicinal herbs, you'll not only enhance your well-being but also deepen your connection to the age-old tradition of harnessing the healing power of plants.

Matching Herbs to Climate Zones:

Selecting and growing herbs that are well-suited to your specific climate zone is a key factor in the success of an herb garden. Herbs, like all plants, have distinct preferences when it comes to temperature, sunlight, and overall climate conditions. Understanding your climate zone and choosing herbs that thrive in that environment will contribute to robust growth, optimal yields, and a flourishing garden. This exploration delves into the considerations for matching herbs to climate zones, offering guidance for successful herb gardening.

Identifying Your Climate Zone:

The first step in matching herbs to climate zones is identifying the specific climate zone of your location. Climate zones are typically categorized based on temperature ranges, and there are various classification systems used globally. The United States, for example, uses the USDA Plant Hardiness Zone Map, which divides the country into zones based on the average annual minimum winter temperature. Understanding your climate zone provides valuable information about the temperature extremes your herbs will face.

Cold-Hardy Herbs for Cooler Climates:

If you are in a cooler climate zone characterized by cold winters, selecting cold-hardy herbs ensures their survival and thriving growth. Herbs such as rosemary, thyme, sage, and chives are known for their resilience in colder temperatures. These herbs can withstand frost and may even benefit from a period of winter dormancy. Providing well-drained soil and protecting them from harsh winter winds enhances their chances of flourishing in cooler climates.

Heat-Tolerant Herbs for Warmer Climates:

In warmer climate zones with hot summers, choosing heat-tolerant herbs is essential for their vitality. Herbs like basil, oregano, mint, and cilantro thrive in warm weather and full sunlight. These herbs not only tolerate higher temperatures but often require warmth to reach their full potential. Providing adequate water and ensuring proper air circulation can further support their growth in hotter climates.

Adaptable Herbs for Variable Climates:

Some regions experience variable or transitional climates, characterized by fluctuations in temperature throughout the year. In such areas, selecting adaptable herbs that can thrive in a range of conditions is beneficial.

Herbs like parsley, dill, and chamomile are known for their adaptability and can endure both cool and warm periods. These versatile herbs can be cultivated across different climate zones with careful attention to their specific needs.

Perennial vs. Annual Herbs:

Consider the life cycle of herbs when matching them to climate zones. Perennial herbs persist through multiple growing seasons, while annual herbs complete their life cycle within a single growing season.

Perennials like thyme, sage, and rosemary may be better suited for climates with mild winters, where they can continue to grow year-round. In contrast, annual herbs like basil and cilantro are well-suited for warmer climates with longer growing seasons.

Microclimates within Your Garden:

Recognize that your garden may contain microclimates—smaller areas with unique temperature and humidity characteristics. Factors such as proximity to walls, bodies of water, or the presence of structures can create microclimates. Observing these variations allows you to strategically place herbs based on their individual preferences, optimizing growing conditions within your garden.

Protecting Herbs from Extreme Conditions:

Extreme weather events, whether cold snaps, heatwaves, or storms, can impact herb gardens. Consider protective measures such as mulching to insulate soil, using row covers during frost events, or providing shade during intense heat. These precautions help mitigate the impact of extreme conditions and support the overall resilience of your herbs.

Local Expertise and Community Insights:

Seek local expertise and insights from gardening communities in your area. Local gardeners often have valuable experience and knowledge about specific herbs that thrive in your climate zone. Attend local gardening events, join online forums, or visit community gardens to tap into the collective wisdom of fellow gardeners who are familiar with the challenges and opportunities of your local climate.

Designing Your Garden Layout

Crafting a garden layout is a creative and rewarding endeavor that involves planning, organization, and a touch of artistic flair.

Whether you're a novice gardener or a seasoned horticulturist, the design of your garden plays a crucial role in its aesthetic appeal, functionality, and overall success. This exploration delves into key considerations for designing your garden layout, offering insights into creating a harmonious green haven that reflects your vision and meets your gardening goals.

Define Your Garden's Purpose:

Before diving into the design process, clearly define the purpose of your garden. Are you cultivating a vegetable garden for sustenance, creating a vibrant flower garden for visual delight, or establishing a medicinal herb garden for holistic well-being? Understanding the primary purpose of your garden informs the layout, plant selection, and overall design elements.

Consider Sunlight and Microclimates:

Assess the sunlight patterns in your garden space, identifying areas with full sun, partial shade, or full shade. Different plants have varying sunlight requirements, and tailoring your garden layout to accommodate these needs is crucial for the health and vitality of your plants. Additionally, observe microclimates within your garden, considering factors such as wind exposure, water drainage, and temperature variations.

Layout Zones for Functionality:

Divide your garden into functional zones based on your gardening activities. Common zones include planting beds, pathways, seating areas, and utility spaces. Designating specific areas for each function creates a well-organized and efficient layout. For example, grouping raised beds for vegetables, herbs, or flowers in one section and reserving another area for relaxation and enjoyment contributes to a functional and visually appealing design.

Create Focal Points and Perspectives:

Introduce focal points and perspectives to add depth and interest to your garden. Consider incorporating eye-catching elements such as a garden sculpture, a water feature, or a striking plant specimen. Establishing focal points creates visual anchors and draws attention to specific areas, enhancing the overall design and creating a sense of balance.

Explore Plant Combinations and Groupings:

Experiment with plant combinations and groupings to create visually stunning arrangements. Consider the colors, textures, and heights of plants when designing your planting beds. Grouping plants with similar water and sunlight requirements not only simplifies maintenance but also fosters a harmonious and cohesive aesthetic. Mixing edible and ornamental plants can add both beauty and functionality to your garden.

Utilize Vertical Space and Layers:

Maximize your garden's potential by utilizing vertical space and creating layers. Vertical gardening, trellises, and arbors not only optimize space but also introduce vertical interest. Incorporate plants with varying heights, from ground covers to tall perennials and shrubs, to create layers that add depth and dimension to your garden design.

Implement Sustainable Practices:

Infuse sustainable practices into your garden layout by incorporating eco-friendly elements. Consider rainwater harvesting, composting, and using native plants that are adapted to your local environment. Embracing sustainable practices not only contributes to environmental stewardship but also enhances the resilience and longevity of your garden.

Plan for Seasonal Interest:

Ensure that your garden offers visual interest throughout the seasons by planning for a succession of blooms, foliage changes, and seasonal features. Select plants with varying bloom times, evergreen specimens for year-round structure, and deciduous trees or shrubs that provide seasonal color. A thoughtfully designed garden provides an ever-changing tapestry of colors and textures.

Balance Hardscape and Softscape Elements:

Achieve a harmonious garden layout by balancing hardscape and softscape elements. Hardscape features such as pathways, borders, and seating areas provide structure, while softscape elements like plants and greenery contribute to a lush and inviting atmosphere. Striking a balance ensures that your garden is both visually appealing and functionally practical.

Adapt the Design to Your Lifestyle:

Tailor your garden layout to align with your lifestyle and preferences. If you enjoy entertaining, create inviting seating areas. If you have a passion for culinary herbs, design a dedicated herb garden near your kitchen. Adapting the design to your lifestyle ensures that your garden becomes a personalized and cherished space.

Companion planting is a centuries-old gardening practice that involves strategically placing different plants in close proximity to enhance each other's growth, deter pests, and maximize overall yield. This age-old technique is rooted in the concept of symbiosis, where certain plants have mutually beneficial relationships when grown together. By understanding the principles of companion planting, gardeners can create harmonious ecosystems that foster healthier plants, reduce the need for chemical interventions, and increase the overall productivity of the garden. This exploration delves into the art and science of companion planting, offering insights into its benefits and popular plant pairings.

1. Biodiversity and Pest Control:

Companion planting contributes to biodiversity in the garden, creating a balanced ecosystem that supports natural pest control. Certain plant combinations work together to repel or confuse pests, reducing the risk of infestations. For example, planting aromatic herbs like basil or rosemary alongside vegetables can deter insect pests, while attracting beneficial insects like ladybugs and predatory wasps that prey on harmful pests.

2. Nutrient Cycling and Soil Health:

Companion planting also plays a role in nutrient cycling and soil health. Different plants have varied nutrient needs, and companion planting helps optimize the use of available nutrients. Legumes, such as peas and beans, have nitrogen-fixing bacteria in their root nodules, enriching the soil with this essential nutrient. Planting nitrogen-loving crops alongside or in rotation with nitrogen-fixing plants promotes a healthy and fertile soil environment.

3. Enhancing Flavor and Aroma:

Certain plant pairings contribute to enhanced flavor and aroma in edible crops. For instance, growing basil near tomatoes is a classic companion planting strategy.

Basil not only deters pests that commonly affect tomatoes but also improves the flavor of the tomatoes. Similarly, planting mint near cabbage family crops can improve the taste of the cabbage while deterring cabbage pests.

4. Space Optimization and Growth Habits:

Companion planting allows for efficient space utilization by taking advantage of different plants' growth habits.

Tall crops can provide shade to more sun-sensitive plants, helping them thrive in warmer climates. Planting compact or trailing varieties near taller plants creates a vertical layering effect, optimizing the use of both horizontal and vertical space in the garden.

5. Trap Cropping and Diversion Tactics:

Strategic companion planting includes the use of trap crops to divert pests away from the main crops. Planting sacrificial crops that are particularly attractive to certain pests can help protect more valuable plants. For example, planting nasturtiums, known to attract aphids, can serve as a trap crop for aphid control in the vicinity of susceptible plants.

6. Three Sisters Planting:

A traditional Native American planting technique known as the "Three Sisters" involves growing corn, beans, and squash together.

This symbiotic trio showcases the principles of companion planting, where the tall corn provides support for the climbing beans, the beans fix nitrogen for the corn, and the squash serves as a ground cover, suppressing weeds and conserving moisture.

7. Allelopathy and Plant Allelochemicals:

Some plants release allelochemicals, compounds that can influence the growth and development of neighboring plants. While allelopathy can be inhibitory in certain cases, it can also be harnessed for positive effects. For example, planting allelopathic crops like marigolds can help suppress weeds and inhibit the growth of certain soil-borne pests.

8. Plant Associations and Traditional Wisdom:

Companion planting draws from traditional wisdom and observations of successful plant associations. Indigenous agricultural practices often incorporate companion planting based on generations of knowledge and experience. Learning from these traditions enriches the repertoire of companion planting strategies and encourages a holistic approach to gardening.

Popular Companion Planting Combinations:

- ➢ Tomatoes and Basil: Basil enhances the flavor of tomatoes and deters pests like aphids and tomato hornworms.
- ➢ Carrots and Onions: Carrots and onions complement each other, with onions deterring carrot flies and carrots repelling onion flies.
- ➢ Cucumbers and Nasturtiums: Nasturtiums serve as a trap crop for aphids, protecting cucumbers, and the trailing nature of nasturtiums provides ground cover.
- ➢ Lettuce and Radishes: Radishes act as a natural pest repellent for lettuce by deterring leaf-eating insects.
- ➢ Beans and Corn: The Three Sisters planting method, where beans climb corn stalks, enriching the soil with nitrogen, and squash serves as a ground cover.

Container Gardening:

Container gardening offers a versatile and accessible way to bring the beauty of plants into spaces with limited ground area, such as balconies, patios, and small yards.

This method of gardening is not only practical for urban dwellers but also provides an opportunity for individuals with varying levels of experience to explore the joys of cultivating flowers, herbs, and even vegetables.

From selecting the right containers to choosing suitable plants, container gardening opens a world of possibilities for creating vibrant and personalized green havens. This exploration delves into the art and benefits of container gardening, offering insights into its diverse applications and tips for success.

1. The Art of Container Selection:

Choosing the right containers is a crucial first step in container gardening. Consider the material, size, and drainage capabilities of the containers.

While clay and ceramic pots are aesthetically pleasing, they may dry out more quickly than plastic or resin containers. Ensure that each container has drainage holes to prevent waterlogged soil, promoting healthy root development. Additionally, match the size of the container to the eventual size of the plants you intend to grow.

2. Soil Matters:

Container plants rely on the potting mix for nutrients, aeration, and drainage. Use a high-quality potting mix that provides a well-balanced blend of organic matter, perlite, and vermiculite. Avoid using garden soil, as it tends to compact in containers, hindering proper drainage and root growth. Consider adding slow-release fertilizer to the potting mix or supplementing with liquid fertilizer throughout the growing season to nourish your container plants.

3. Plant Selection and Arrangement:

Container gardening allows for a wide range of plant choices, including flowers, herbs, vegetables, and even small trees or shrubs. Consider the growing conditions of your space, such as sunlight exposure and microclimates, when selecting plants. Mix and match plants with similar water and sunlight requirements, and pay attention to their growth habits. Taller plants can provide vertical interest, while trailing or compact varieties add texture and depth.

4. Watering Wisdom:

Proper watering is a key to success in container gardening. Containers can dry out more quickly than garden beds, especially during hot weather. Establish a regular watering routine and monitor the moisture levels of the potting mix. Water thoroughly until water drains from the bottom of the container, ensuring that the entire root zone is adequately hydrated. Consider using self-watering containers or incorporating moisture-retaining materials like mulch to reduce water evaporation.

5. Sunlight and Placement:

Understanding the sunlight requirements of your chosen plants is essential for successful container gardening. Most flowering plants, herbs, and vegetables thrive in full sunlight, while some may tolerate partial shade. Observe the sunlight patterns in your space and place containers accordingly. Consider the versatility of containers, allowing you to move them to optimal locations as the seasons change or as sunlight conditions evolve.

6. Creative Container Arrangements:

Container gardening invites creativity in arranging plants to create visually appealing compositions. Experiment with different color combinations, textures, and heights to design containers that complement each other and enhance your overall outdoor space. Mixing ornamental plants with edible herbs or vegetables adds both visual interest and functionality to your container arrangements.

7. Seasonal Refresh and Succession Planting:

Embrace the changing seasons by refreshing your container displays to suit the time of year. Consider incorporating seasonal flowers, such as pansies in the spring or chrysanthemums in the fall, to celebrate the beauty of each season. Additionally, practice succession planting by replacing spent crops with new ones, ensuring a continuous harvest and vibrant container displays throughout the growing season.

8. Vertical Gardening with Containers:

Take advantage of vertical space by incorporating hanging baskets, wall-mounted containers, or vertical planters. Vertical gardening not only maximizes space but also adds an artistic dimension to your container garden. Consider trailing plants like petunias or ivy for hanging containers and compact varieties for vertical planters.

9. Pest Management in Containers:

Container gardening can help mitigate certain pest issues, but it's essential to stay vigilant. Check plants regularly for signs of pests, such as aphids or spider mites, and address any issues promptly. Consider using companion planting strategies, such as planting marigolds to deter nematodes, to naturally reduce the risk of pest infestations.

10. Overwintering and Storage:

In regions with harsh winters, consider the overwintering needs of your container plants. Some plants may be hardy enough to survive outdoors, while others may benefit from winter protection. Move containers to sheltered areas, wrap them in insulating material, or place them in unheated garages or sheds to protect them from extreme cold. Container gardening offers a wealth of possibilities for individuals with varying levels of gardening experience and limited outdoor space.

Whether you're cultivating a colorful display of flowers, a collection of culinary herbs, or a small vegetable garden, containers provide a platform for creativity and experimentation. By paying attention to the unique needs of container plants and embracing the flexibility that containers offer, you can create a thriving and personalized green oasis that brings joy and natural beauty to your urban or small-space living.

Seeds vs. Seedlings

Starting your medicinal herb garden can be an exciting venture, but one of the key decisions you'll face is whether to begin with seeds or seedlings. Each method has its own set of advantages and challenges, and understanding the nuances can greatly impact the success of your herb-growing journey.

Seeds: The Beginning of Life

Embarking on the journey of growing medicinal herbs from seeds is a fulfilling and educational experience. It's a process that allows you to witness the entire life cycle of a plant, from germination to maturity. When choosing seeds, you open the door to a wide variety of herb species and cultivars that might not be readily available as seedlings. This diversity provides the opportunity to cultivate unique and specialized herbs tailored to your specific health and wellness needs.

Starting from seeds also gives you greater control over the growing conditions right from the beginning. You can choose organic, non-GMO seeds and create an environment that minimizes the risk of introducing pests or diseases. The germination phase, while requiring patience, is a fascinating stage where you witness the emergence of life from a tiny seed. It's a process that connects you intimately with the plants you're nurturing.

However, it's important to note that growing herbs from seeds demands careful attention and commitment. You'll need to provide the optimal conditions for germination, including the right temperature, humidity, and light. Some herbs may have specific germination requirements, such as stratification or scarification, which adds an extra layer of complexity to the process. Additionally, the time it takes for herbs to grow from seeds to mature plants can be longer compared to starting with seedlings.

Seedlings: A Head Start to Your Garden

Opting for seedlings offers a more convenient and time-saving approach to establishing your medicinal herb garden. Seedlings are young plants that have already passed the delicate germination stage and have developed a basic root and shoot structure. Choosing seedlings provides you with a head start, allowing you to enjoy mature herbs more quickly and harvest your medicinal plants sooner.

One of the main advantages of starting with seedlings is the reduced time and effort required to get your garden up and running. Seedlings have already overcome the vulnerable early stages, and you can skip the germination phase, which can be challenging for beginners. This method is particularly beneficial if you have a shorter growing season or if you're eager to enjoy the medicinal benefits of herbs sooner rather than later.

However, purchasing seedlings might limit your selection of herb varieties, as nurseries may offer a more limited range compared to the vast options available through seeds. Additionally, there's the potential risk of introducing pests or diseases if you're not diligent in inspecting and quarantining your seedlings before transplanting them into your garden.

Whether you choose to start your medicinal herb garden from seeds or seedlings depends on your preferences, available time, and level of expertise. Each method has its own unique set of rewards and challenges, and the decision ultimately comes down to what aligns with your goals and gardening style. Whichever path you choose, the journey of cultivating medicinal herbs is a fulfilling and enriching experience that connects you with the therapeutic wonders of nature.

Germination Tips

Germination marks the commencement of a plant's life cycle, a pivotal stage in the journey of cultivating medicinal herbs. Whether you're a novice gardener or an experienced herbalist, understanding and mastering germination is crucial for a successful herb garden. Here are some essential germination tips to guide you through this fundamental phase.

1. Selecting Quality Seeds:

The germination process begins with the seed, making it imperative to start with high-quality, viable seeds. Opt for reputable seed suppliers to ensure the seeds are fresh, disease-free, and genetically sound. Check for the seed's packaging date, as fresher seeds generally have higher germination rates. Investing in quality seeds lays a strong foundation for successful germination and healthy plant development.

2. Understanding Germination Requirements:

Different herbs have varying germination requirements, influenced by factors like temperature, light, moisture, and soil type. Research the specific needs of each herb you intend to grow, as understanding these requirements is key to fostering optimal germination conditions.

Some seeds may require stratification (a period of cold treatment), while others may need scarification (scratching or breaking the seed coat) to enhance germination. Tailoring your approach to each herb's unique needs increases the likelihood of successful germination.

3. Providing the Right Growing Medium:

The choice of a suitable growing medium significantly impacts germination success. Use a well-draining and sterile seed-starting mix to prevent diseases and provide an environment conducive to root development. A mix of peat, vermiculite, and perlite is a popular choice for starting seeds. Ensure the growing medium is consistently moist but not waterlogged, striking a balance that facilitates the absorption of water by the seeds without suffocating them.

4. Temperature Control:

Temperature plays a critical role in germination, influencing the speed and success of the process. Most herbs prefer warm soil for germination. Consider using a heat mat to maintain a consistent temperature, especially if you're germinating seeds indoors or in a cooler climate. Germination typically occurs faster when the soil temperature is within the ideal range for each herb, fostering the activation of enzymes that kickstart the growth process.

5. Adequate Moisture:

Maintaining optimal moisture levels is essential for successful germination. Seeds need moisture to soften their protective coats and initiate the germination process. However, excess moisture can lead to fungal issues and damping off. Use a fine mist sprayer or a humidity dome to create a humid environment during the germination phase. Once the seedlings emerge, gradually reduce humidity to prevent fungal problems and encourage sturdy plant growth.

6. Light Conditions:

While some seeds require darkness for germination, most herb seeds benefit from exposure to light. Ensure you follow the specific light requirements of the herbs you're cultivating. If light is necessary, provide gentle, indirect light to prevent stressing the emerging seedlings. Using fluorescent or LED grow lights can be beneficial, especially when germinating seeds indoors or during cloudy periods.

7. Patience and Observation:

Germination is a process that demands patience and keen observation. Different herbs have varied germination times, ranging from a few days to several weeks. Regularly check the trays or pots for signs of emerging seedlings, adjusting conditions as needed. Be prepared for variations in germination times among different herb species, and avoid the temptation to disturb the seeds or seedlings unnecessarily.

8. Thinning Seedlings:

As seedlings emerge, resist the urge to overcrowd the growing space. Thinning, or removing excess seedlings, is a crucial step to ensure proper airflow and prevent competition for nutrients. Gently thin the seedlings, leaving only the strongest and healthiest individuals. This practice contributes to robust plant development and reduces the risk of disease.

9. Transplanting Seedlings:

Once your seedlings have developed a strong root system and a few sets of true leaves, they are ready for transplantation. Handle seedlings carefully, holding them by their leaves to avoid damage to the delicate stems. Transplant the seedlings into larger containers or directly into the garden, taking care to acclimate them gradually to outdoor conditions if they were started indoors.

10. Record-Keeping:

Maintaining a gardening journal can significantly contribute to your success in germination and overall herb cultivation. Record details such as seed varieties, germination dates, and any observations about the process. This valuable information serves as a reference for future planting seasons, helping you refine your techniques and enhance your gardening skills.

Successful germination is a vital step in the journey of growing medicinal herbs. By carefully selecting quality seeds, understanding germination requirements, providing an ideal growing medium, controlling temperature and moisture, ensuring adequate light, exercising patience, thinning seedlings, and practicing diligent record-keeping, you set the stage for a thriving herb garden. Mastering the art of germination not only fosters healthy plant development but also deepens your connection with the intricate and awe-inspiring process of life emerging from a tiny seed.

Embarking on the journey of growing medicinal herbs from seeds is a rewarding endeavor that begins with a crucial step: purchasing quality seeds. The success of your herb garden hinges on the vitality and reliability of the seeds you choose. Here are key considerations and tips to guide you when selecting seeds for your medicinal herb garden.

1. Research and Choose Reputable Suppliers:

The foundation of obtaining quality seeds lies in choosing reputable suppliers. Research and identify well-established seed companies or nurseries known for their commitment to providing reliable, high-quality seeds. Reading customer reviews and seeking recommendations from experienced gardeners can help you gauge the reputation and reliability of potential suppliers.

2. Opt for Organic and Non-GMO Seeds:

For a truly holistic approach to medicinal herb cultivation, opt for organic and non-genetically modified organism (GMO) seeds. Organic seeds are produced without synthetic pesticides or fertilizers, aligning with a natural and sustainable gardening ethos. Non-GMO seeds ensure that the genetic integrity of the plants remains unaltered, preserving the natural characteristics and potential health benefits of the herbs.

3. Check Seed Packaging Information:

Examine the information provided on the seed packaging. Look for details such as the seed's botanical name, germination rate, and any specific instructions or requirements for successful cultivation. High-quality seed packages often include valuable information about the plant's characteristics, growing conditions, and potential uses, aiding in informed decision-making.

4. Consider Seed Viability and Freshness:

The viability and freshness of seeds are critical factors in successful germination. Check the packaging date or the seed's expiration date to ensure you are purchasing fresh seeds. Fresh seeds generally have higher germination rates, increasing the likelihood of successful plant establishment. When possible, choose seeds from the most recent harvest to maximize their vitality.

5. Understand Seed Varieties and Cultivars:

Medicinal herbs come in various varieties and cultivars, each with its unique traits and properties. Understand the specific varieties and cultivars of the herbs you intend to grow, as this knowledge influences the selection of seeds. Some herbs may have multiple cultivars with variations in flavor, aroma, or medicinal compounds. Choose seeds that align with your preferences and intended use of the herbs.

6. Check for Disease Resistance:

Disease-resistant seeds can be invaluable in preventing potential issues in your herb garden. While no seeds guarantee complete immunity, some varieties have been bred for increased resistance to common diseases. Check for information on disease resistance when selecting seeds, especially if you are cultivating herbs in conditions prone to specific diseases.

7. Explore Heirloom Seeds:

Heirloom seeds are open-pollinated varieties that have been passed down through generations, preserving their unique characteristics. Choosing heirloom seeds not only contributes to biodiversity but also allows you to grow plants with historical significance. Additionally, heirloom varieties often boast distinct flavors and traits, enhancing the diversity and richness of your medicinal herb garden.

8. Consider Your Growing Conditions:

Take into account your local climate, soil type, and growing conditions when selecting seeds. Some herbs thrive in specific climates or soil types, and choosing seeds adapted to your local conditions increases the likelihood of successful cultivation. Check the hardiness zone recommendations on the seed packaging to ensure compatibility with your region.

9. Look for Seed Certification:

Seed certification indicates that the seeds meet certain quality standards and have undergone testing for purity and germination rates. Certified seeds have been inspected by relevant authorities to ensure they adhere to specific guidelines. While not all quality seeds are certified, this designation can provide an extra layer of assurance regarding the seed's quality and reliability.

10. Budget Considerations:

While it's important to prioritize quality, consider your budget when purchasing seeds. Quality seeds may come with a higher price tag, but the investment is often worthwhile for a successful and bountiful herb garden. Balance your budget constraints with the long-term benefits of cultivating high-quality medicinal herbs.

Purchasing quality seeds is a foundational step in the journey of growing medicinal herbs. By researching reputable suppliers, choosing organic and non-GMO seeds, checking seed packaging information, considering viability and freshness, understanding seed varieties, checking for disease resistance, exploring heirloom options, considering local growing conditions, looking for seed certification, and balancing your budget, you set the stage for a flourishing and sustainable herb garden. The careful selection of seeds not only ensures a successful start but also contributes to the overall health and vitality of your medicinal herb plants.

Soil Preparation and Fertilization

Creating the ideal environment for your medicinal herb garden starts with thoughtful soil preparation and strategic fertilization. These foundational practices not only contribute to the overall health of your plants but also play a crucial role in maximizing the medicinal properties of the herbs you cultivate. Here are key considerations and tips for effective soil preparation and fertilization in your medicinal herb garden.

1. Soil Testing:

Before diving into soil preparation, conduct a thorough soil test to understand the composition and pH of your soil. Soil testing provides valuable insights into nutrient levels, potential deficiencies, and acidity or alkalinity. Armed with this information, you can tailor your soil preparation and fertilization strategies to address specific needs, creating an optimal growing environment for your medicinal herbs.

2. Organic Matter and Soil Structure:

Incorporating organic matter into your soil is fundamental for creating a nutrient-rich and well-structured growing medium. Compost, well-rotted manure, and other organic amendments enhance soil structure, promoting good drainage and aeration. This is particularly important for medicinal herbs, as many prefer well-draining soil to prevent waterlogged conditions, which can lead to root rot and other issues.

3. Choosing the Right Soil Mix:

Different medicinal herbs have varying soil preferences. Some thrive in well-drained, sandy soils, while others prefer loamy or slightly acidic conditions. Tailor your soil mix to match the specific requirements of the herbs you're cultivating. Adding perlite or vermiculite can improve drainage, and incorporating organic matter helps retain moisture and nutrients.

4. pH Adjustment:

Soil pH profoundly influences nutrient availability to plants. Most medicinal herbs prefer a slightly acidic to neutral pH range. Adjusting soil pH can be necessary, especially if your soil tends to be too alkaline or acidic. Limestone can be added to raise pH, while elemental sulfur or acidic organic materials like pine needles can lower it. Regular monitoring and adjustment of pH contribute to the overall health and vitality of your medicinal herb garden.

5. Fertilizing with Natural Nutrients:

Fertilization is a key aspect of soil preparation, providing essential nutrients to support the growth and development of medicinal herbs. Opt for natural, organic fertilizers that contribute to the overall health of the soil ecosystem. Compost, well-rotted manure, and organic blends enrich the soil with a balanced mix of nutrients and foster beneficial microbial activity.

6. Timing and Application Rates:

Timing and application rates are crucial aspects of effective fertilization. Apply fertilizers at the right stage of plant growth, ensuring that nutrients are available when the herbs need them most. Over-fertilization can lead to nutrient imbalances and environmental concerns, so follow recommended application rates and schedule fertilization based on the specific needs of your medicinal herbs.

7. Slow-Release Fertilizers:

Consider incorporating slow-release fertilizers into your soil preparation routine. These formulations provide a steady, gradual release of nutrients over an extended period, promoting sustained growth and reducing the risk of nutrient leaching. Slow-release fertilizers are particularly beneficial for medicinal herbs, as they align with the plants' natural growth patterns and reduce the need for frequent applications.

8. Companion Planting for Natural Fertilization:

Explore the concept of companion planting as a natural method of fertilization. Certain plant combinations can enhance nutrient uptake, deter pests, and create a harmonious growing environment. For example, planting nitrogen-fixing legumes alongside medicinal herbs can contribute nitrogen to the soil, enriching it naturally. Research companion planting strategies that align with the preferences of your medicinal herbs.

9. Mulching: Preserving Soil Moisture and Nutrients

Mulching serves as a multifaceted technique in soil preparation and fertilization. Applying a layer of organic mulch, such as straw or shredded leaves, helps retain soil moisture, suppress weeds, and gradually release nutrients as the mulch breaks down. Mulching also insulates the soil, providing a buffer against temperature extremes and promoting a favorable environment for soil-dwelling organisms.

10. Sustainable Practices: Nurturing the Soil for Future Growth

Adopt sustainable practices in your soil preparation and fertilization routines to ensure the long-term health of your medicinal herb garden. Rotate crops to prevent nutrient depletion and minimize the risk of soil-borne diseases. Practice water conservation to maintain soil structure and microbial activity. Embrace organic and eco-friendly fertilization methods, minimizing the impact on the environment.

Soil preparation and fertilization are fundamental pillars of successful medicinal herb cultivation. By conducting soil tests, incorporating organic matter, customizing soil mixes, adjusting pH, choosing natural fertilizers, timing applications, embracing slow-release options, exploring companion planting, implementing mulching, and adopting sustainable practices, you establish a nurturing environment for your medicinal herbs to thrive. These practices not only support immediate growth but also contribute to the long-term vitality of your medicinal herb garden, ensuring a bountiful harvest of potent and health-promoting herbs.

Organic Soil Amendments

Organic soil amendments are the backbone of sustainable and environmentally friendly gardening practices. Choosing natural, organic materials to enhance the fertility and structure of your soil is a fundamental aspect of cultivating a thriving and healthy medicinal herb garden. Here, we explore the importance of organic soil amendments and highlight some key options for enriching your soil naturally.

1. Building Soil Structure with Compost:

Compost is often referred to as "black gold" in gardening, and for good reason. This nutrient-rich organic matter is a powerhouse when it comes to enhancing soil structure. Compost improves both drainage and water retention, creating a well-balanced environment for medicinal herbs. It also introduces a diverse array of beneficial microorganisms that contribute to the soil's overall health. As compost breaks down, it releases essential nutrients, providing a slow and steady supply to your plants.

2. Well-Rotted Manure for Nutrient Boost:

Well-rotted manure, derived from herbivores such as cows, horses, or chickens, is an excellent source of organic matter and essential nutrients. When properly composted, manure undergoes a transformation that reduces the risk of pathogens and weed seeds. Incorporating well-rotted manure into your soil adds nitrogen, phosphorus, and potassium—key nutrients for plant growth. This natural fertilizer contributes to the overall fertility of the soil, promoting robust and vigorous medicinal herbs.

3. Harnessing the Power of Worm Castings:

Worm castings, often referred to as "black gold" like compost, are a nutrient-dense organic amendment produced by earthworms. These castings are rich in beneficial microorganisms, enzymes, and plant-available nutrients. Worm castings improve soil structure, enhance water retention, and contribute to increased nutrient absorption by plants. Incorporating worm castings into your soil not only provides immediate benefits but also establishes a thriving ecosystem within the soil.

4. Cover Crops for Green Manure:

Cover crops, also known as green manure, serve a dual purpose in organic gardening. These crops are planted to cover and protect the soil during periods when the main crop isn't growing. When the cover crop is eventually incorporated into the soil, it adds organic matter, suppresses weeds, and enhances fertility. Leguminous cover crops, such as clover or vetch, have the added benefit of fixing nitrogen from the air into the soil, enriching it naturally.

5. Seaweed and Kelp: A Boost of Minerals:

Seaweed and kelp are excellent organic soil amendments that bring a wealth of trace minerals to your garden. These marine plants are not only rich in micronutrients but also contain hormones that stimulate plant growth.

Seaweed can be applied directly to the soil or used to make a nutrient-rich tea. When used as a foliar spray, it provides a quick and efficient way for plants to absorb the benefits of these mineral-rich amendments.

6. Bone Meal and Fish Emulsion for Phosphorus and Nitrogen:

Bone meal, a byproduct of the meat industry, is a valuable organic amendment high in phosphorus. Phosphorus is essential for root development and overall plant energy transfer. Fish emulsion, derived from fish waste, is an excellent source of nitrogen. Nitrogen is a vital nutrient for leafy green growth. Both bone meal and fish emulsion provide slow-release nutrients to the soil, supporting the specific needs of different medicinal herbs.

7. Wood Ash for Potassium and Adjusting pH:

Wood ash, a byproduct of burning wood, can be used as an organic amendment to supply potassium and raise soil pH. Potassium is crucial for overall plant health, contributing to disease resistance and water uptake. However, it's important to use wood ash sparingly, as excessive amounts can increase soil alkalinity. Regular soil testing is recommended to monitor pH levels and ensure a balanced environment for your medicinal herbs.

8. Alfalfa Meal: A Multi-Benefit Amendment:

Alfalfa meal is a versatile organic amendment that provides multiple benefits to the soil. It contains nitrogen, phosphorus, potassium, and various trace minerals. Additionally, alfalfa contains triacontanol, a natural growth stimulant. When added to the soil, alfalfa meal improves fertility, encourages beneficial microorganisms, and enhances overall plant vigor. Its slow-release nature makes it a sustainable choice for long-term soil enrichment.

9. Bat Guano: A Natural Fertilizer:

Bat guano, derived from bat excrement, is a potent and natural fertilizer rich in nitrogen, phosphorus, and potassium. It is known for its high nutrient content and the absence of odor, making it a convenient option for organic gardening. Bat guano can be applied to the soil or used as a component in compost teas to provide a nutrient boost for your medicinal herbs.

10. Eggshells for Calcium:

Eggshells, often discarded as waste, can be repurposed as a valuable organic soil amendment. Crushed eggshells add calcium to the soil, which is essential for cell division, enzyme activation, and overall plant structure. In addition to providing a slow-release source of calcium, eggshells can help deter certain pests, such as snails and slugs, due to their abrasive texture.

Organic soil amendments are essential for creating a nutrient-rich, well-structured, and sustainable environment for your medicinal herb garden. By incorporating compost, well-rotted manure, worm castings, cover crops, seaweed, kelp, bone meal, fish emulsion, wood ash, alfalfa meal, bat guano, eggshells, and other natural materials, you not only nourish your plants but also foster a thriving ecosystem within the soil. These organic practices contribute to the long-term health of your medicinal herbs, ensuring a bountiful harvest of potent and beneficial plants.

Fertilizing Techniques

Fertilizing is a critical aspect of cultivating a successful and productive medicinal herb garden. The application of nutrients through fertilization provides essential elements for plant growth, health, and the development of medicinal compounds. Understanding and implementing effective fertilizing techniques are key to maximizing the potential of your herbs. Here, we delve into various fertilizing techniques to help you nurture a thriving medicinal herb garden.

1. Soil Testing for Precision:

Before initiating any fertilizing regimen, conduct a soil test to assess the nutrient levels and pH of your soil. Soil testing provides valuable insights into specific deficiencies or excesses, allowing you to tailor your fertilizing approach. Understanding your soil's unique composition ensures that you provide the right nutrients in the right amounts, optimizing the overall health of your medicinal herbs.

2. Balanced and Complete Fertilizers:

Choosing a balanced and complete fertilizer is a foundational step in effective fertilizing. Look for organic or slow-release fertilizers that contain a mix of essential nutrients, including nitrogen (N), phosphorus (P), and ptassium (K). These primary nutrients support different aspects of plant growth, with nitrogen promoting leafy growth, phosphorus aiding in root development, and potassium contributing to overall plant health and disease resistance.

3. Timing Matters:

The timing of fertilization plays a crucial role in the success of your medicinal herb garden. Apply fertilizers at the right stage of plant growth to meet the specific needs of your herbs. For instance, nitrogen-rich fertilizers are beneficial during the vegetative growth phase, while phosphorus becomes more critical during flowering and fruiting. Understanding the growth cycles of your medicinal herbs helps you time fertilizer applications for maximum impact.

4. Foliar Feeding:

Foliar feeding involves applying liquid fertilizer directly to the leaves of your plants. This technique allows for rapid nutrient absorption, especially in instances where the soil may be deficient or if the plants require a quick nutrient boost. Create a nutrient-rich solution and spray it on the foliage, ensuring thorough coverage. Foliar feeding is particularly useful for addressing immediate nutrient deficiencies or promoting faster growth during crucial stages.

5. Top-Dressing with Compost:

Top-dressing with compost is a simple yet effective fertilizing technique that enhances soil fertility and structure. Spread a layer of well-aged compost around the base of your medicinal herbs, avoiding direct contact with stems. This top-dressing not only provides a slow-release source of nutrients but also introduces beneficial microorganisms to the soil, promoting a healthy and thriving ecosystem.

6. Incorporating Organic Amendments:

Organic amendments, such as well-rotted manure, bone meal, or fish emulsion, contribute to the overall fertility of the soil. These amendments release nutrients gradually, providing a sustained source of nourishment for your medicinal herbs. Incorporate organic amendments into the soil during the growing season or as part of your initial soil preparation, ensuring a well-balanced and nutrient-rich environment.

7. Utilizing Controlled-Release Fertilizers:

Controlled-release or slow-release fertilizers offer a convenient and efficient way to provide nutrients to your medicinal herbs over an extended period. These granular or pelletized fertilizers release nutrients gradually in response to environmental factors such as temperature and moisture. Controlled-release fertilizers are especially beneficial for those who prefer a low-maintenance approach to fertilizing, providing a steady supply of nutrients without the need for frequent applications.

8. Companion Planting for Natural Nutrient Exchange:

Companion planting involves strategically placing plants with mutually beneficial relationships in close proximity. Some plants naturally complement each other by exchanging nutrients or deterring pests. Utilize companion planting techniques to enhance nutrient exchange in your medicinal herb garden. For example, planting nitrogen-fixing legumes alongside other herbs can contribute nitrogen to the soil, benefiting neighboring plants.

9. Drip Irrigation with Fertilizer Injection:

Drip irrigation systems with fertilizer injection offer a precise and efficient method of delivering nutrients directly to the root zone. This automated system ensures uniform distribution of fertilizers, minimizing waste and optimizing nutrient uptake by your medicinal herbs. Fertilizer injectors can be adjusted to meet the specific needs of different herbs, providing a customizable and controlled approach to fertilizing.

10. Adjusting Nutrient Ratios Based on Herb Preferences:

Different medicinal herbs have varied nutrient requirements based on their growth characteristics and intended use. Research the specific needs of each herb in your garden and adjust nutrient ratios accordingly.

Customizing your fertilizing approach to match the preferences of your medicinal herbs promotes optimal growth, enhances medicinal compound development, and ensures a harvest of potent and health-promoting plants. Effective fertilizing techniques are essential for cultivating a flourishing medicinal herb garden.

By conducting soil tests, choosing balanced and complete fertilizers, timing applications strategically, incorporating organic amendments, utilizing controlled-release fertilizers, practicing foliar feeding, top-dressing with compost, exploring companion planting, adopting drip irrigation with fertilizer injection, and adjusting nutrient ratios based on herb preferences, you create a nutrient-rich and well-balanced environment for your herbs to thrive. These techniques not only support immediate growth but also contribute to the long-term health and potency of your medicinal herb garden.

Watering and irrigation are fundamental aspects of maintaining a healthy and thriving medicinal herb garden. Providing an adequate and consistent water supply is crucial for the growth, development, and medicinal potency of the herbs.

Proper watering techniques, combined with efficient irrigation practices, contribute to the overall success of your garden. Here, we explore key considerations and tips for effective watering and irrigation in your medicinal herb garden.

1. Understanding Herb Water Requirements:

Different medicinal herbs have varying water needs based on their natural habitat and growth characteristics. Conduct thorough research on the specific water requirements of each herb in your garden. Some herbs prefer consistently moist soil, while others thrive in well-drained conditions. Understanding these preferences enables you to tailor your watering and irrigation practices to meet the individual needs of each plant.

2. Soil Moisture Monitoring:

Regularly monitor soil moisture levels to gauge when and how much water your medicinal herbs need. Use a soil moisture meter or perform a simple finger test to assess soil moisture. Insert your finger into the soil up to the second knuckle; if it feels dry at that depth, it's time to water. Monitoring soil moisture helps prevent both under-watering, which can lead to stress and reduced growth, and over-watering, which may result in root rot and other issues.

3. Watering at the Right Time:

Timing is crucial when it comes to watering your medicinal herbs. Water early in the day to allow the foliage to dry before evening, reducing the risk of fungal diseases. Morning watering also ensures that plants are adequately hydrated for the day ahead. Avoid watering in the heat of the afternoon, as rapid evaporation may limit the absorption of water by the plants.

4. Deep and Infrequent Watering:

Encourage deep root development by practicing deep and infrequent watering. This technique promotes strong and resilient root systems, making your medicinal herbs more resistant to drought conditions.

Water deeply to saturate the root zone, and then allow the soil to dry out before the next watering. This approach encourages roots to seek moisture at deeper levels, contributing to the overall health of the plants.

5. Mulching for Moisture Retention:

Mulching is a valuable practice for conserving soil moisture and regulating temperature. Apply a layer of organic mulch, such as straw, wood chips, or shredded leaves, around the base of your medicinal herbs. Mulch acts as a protective barrier, reducing water evaporation, suppressing weeds, and maintaining a more consistent soil temperature. This, in turn, minimizes the frequency of watering while ensuring a more efficient use of water.

6. Drip Irrigation for Precision:

Drip irrigation is a precise and efficient method of delivering water directly to the root zone of your medicinal herbs. This system minimizes water waste by avoiding overhead watering, which can lead to evaporation and foliar diseases. Drip irrigation also helps maintain soil structure by preventing compaction caused by traditional watering methods. Adjust the flow rate to match the water needs of different herbs, providing a customized and controlled watering solution.

7. Rain Barrels for Sustainable Watering:

Incorporate rain barrels into your irrigation system to harness and store rainwater for garden use. Rainwater is naturally soft and free from chlorine and other additives found in tap water. Using rain barrels not only conserves water but also provides your medicinal herbs with a more natural and beneficial water source. Position rain barrels strategically to capture runoff from roofs and gutters.

8. Monitoring Environmental Conditions:

Pay attention to environmental factors that may influence watering needs. Hot and windy conditions can increase evaporation rates, requiring more frequent watering. Conversely, periods of high humidity may necessitate less frequent watering. Adjust your watering schedule based on the specific conditions in your garden, taking into account temperature, humidity, and rainfall patterns.

9. Proper Container Watering:

If you're growing medicinal herbs in containers, be mindful of their unique watering requirements. Containers tend to dry out more quickly than garden beds, so monitor soil moisture regularly.

Water thoroughly until you see water draining from the bottom of the container, ensuring that the entire root ball is adequately hydrated. Consider using potting mixes with water-retaining additives for container gardening.

10. Conserving Water with Smart Practices:

Embrace water conservation practices in your medicinal herb garden to minimize waste and promote sustainability. Collect rainwater, reuse greywater when feasible, and implement smart irrigation technologies that optimize water use. Grouping plants with similar water needs together can also streamline watering efforts, ensuring that each herb receives the appropriate amount of moisture.

Effective watering and irrigation practices are integral to the success of your medicinal herb garden. By understanding the water requirements of individual herbs, monitoring soil moisture, timing watering appropriately, practicing deep and infrequent watering, using mulch for moisture retention, implementing drip irrigation for precision, incorporating rain barrels for sustainability, adjusting watering based on environmental conditions, and adopting proper container watering techniques, you create a conducive environment for the optimal growth and medicinal potency of your herbs. These techniques not only promote the health and vitality of your medicinal herb garden but also contribute to sustainable and water-efficient gardening practices.

Watering Schedule

Establishing a well-thought-out watering schedule is a crucial component of successful medicinal herb gardening. Adequate and consistent hydration is essential for the growth, development, and medicinal potency of herbs. Crafting a watering schedule that aligns with the specific needs of your medicinal plants ensures optimal health and resilience. Here, we delve into key considerations and tips for creating an effective watering schedule for your medicinal herb garden.

1. Know Your Herbs:

The foundation of a successful watering schedule lies in understanding the specific water requirements of each medicinal herb in your garden. Different herbs have varying preferences based on factors such as their native habitats, growth habits, and leaf structures. Research the individual needs of your herbs to tailor your watering schedule accordingly. For example, herbs originating from arid regions may prefer drier conditions, while those from humid environments may thrive with more frequent watering.

2. Consider Soil Type and Drainage:

The type of soil in your garden greatly influences its water-holding capacity and drainage. Sandy soils drain quickly but may require more frequent watering, while clay soils retain water but can become waterlogged if not adequately drained. Adjust your watering schedule based on the soil type, incorporating practices like amending with organic matter to improve water retention or adding drainage amendments for better soil structure.

3. Morning Watering for Plant Health:

Timing matters when it comes to watering your medicinal herbs. The morning is generally the ideal time for watering as it allows the foliage to dry before evening, minimizing the risk of fungal diseases. Morning watering ensures that plants are hydrated and ready to face the day, promoting overall plant health and resilience.

4. Deep and Infrequent Watering:

Encourage robust root development by practicing deep and infrequent watering. This technique involves providing a substantial amount of water at each watering session, saturating the root zone. Allow the soil to dry out between watering to promote the development of a resilient root system that can better withstand drought conditions. Deep and infrequent watering encourages roots to grow deeper, accessing moisture at lower soil levels.

5. Adjust Watering Frequency Based on Season:

Seasonal changes significantly impact the water requirements of your medicinal herbs. During hotter months, when evaporation rates are high, you may need to increase the frequency of watering. In contrast, cooler seasons may require less frequent watering. Stay attuned to seasonal variations and adjust your watering schedule accordingly, ensuring that your herbs receive the appropriate amount of moisture throughout the year.

6. Monitor Soil Moisture Regularly:

Regular monitoring of soil moisture is essential for fine-tuning your watering schedule. Use a soil moisture meter or perform a simple finger test by checking the soil's moisture content at different depths. If the soil feels dry at the top but moist deeper down, it may not be time to water. Regular monitoring helps you avoid over-watering, a common issue that can lead to root rot and other problems.

7. Tailor Watering to Container Plants:

If you're growing medicinal herbs in containers, adapt your watering schedule to the unique needs of potted plants. Containers tend to dry out more quickly than garden beds, so check the soil moisture in containers more frequently. Adjust your watering schedule for potted herbs based on the specific conditions, taking into account factors such as container size, type of potting mix, and exposure to sunlight.

8. Mulching for Moisture Retention:

Mulching is an effective practice for conserving soil moisture and regulating temperature. Apply a layer of organic mulch around the base of your medicinal herbs to reduce water evaporation, suppress weeds, and maintain a more even soil temperature. Mulching helps extend the time between watering sessions, providing a buffer against fluctuations in soil moisture.

9. Watering Newly Planted Herbs:

Newly planted herbs require special attention in terms of watering. Initially, these herbs may need more frequent watering to establish their root systems. As the plants mature and roots expand, gradually adjust the watering schedule to promote deep root growth. Be mindful not to over-water newly planted herbs, as this can hinder the development of a robust root system.

10. Use Watering Tools Wisely:

Selecting the right watering tools contributes to the effectiveness of your watering schedule. Consider using a soaker hose or drip irrigation system for precise and controlled watering, especially in larger gardens.

These tools minimize water waste and ensure that moisture reaches the root zone where it's needed most. Hand watering with a gentle nozzle can be beneficial for smaller or container gardens, providing a personal touch to your care routine.

Crafting a well-defined watering schedule is essential for nurturing a thriving medicinal herb garden. By understanding the unique water requirements of your herbs, considering soil type and drainage, timing watering sessions appropriately, practicing deep and infrequent watering, adjusting frequency based on season, monitoring soil moisture regularly, tailoring watering to container plants, mulching for moisture retention, watering newly planted herbs with care, and using watering tools wisely, you create an environment that promotes optimal growth and medicinal potency.

A thoughtful watering schedule not only supports the immediate health of your medicinal herbs but also contributes to the long-term sustainability of your garden.

Avoiding Common Mistakes

Cultivating a successful medicinal herb garden can be a rewarding journey, but it's not without its challenges. To ensure the health, vitality, and potency of your herbs, it's crucial to be aware of common mistakes that gardeners may inadvertently make. By understanding and avoiding these pitfalls, you can set the stage for a flourishing herb garden. Here, we explore some key mistakes to avoid in your medicinal herb cultivation.

1. Lack of Research:

One of the most common mistakes is diving into herb gardening without sufficient research. Each medicinal herb has unique requirements regarding sunlight, soil type, water, and nutrients. Failure to understand these specific needs can lead to poor growth, reduced medicinal properties, and even the loss of plants. Take the time to thoroughly research each herb you intend to grow, considering factors such as its native habitat, growth habits, and potential challenges.

2. Overcrowding Plants:

Overcrowding is a frequent mistake, particularly for enthusiastic beginners eager to cultivate a diverse herb garden. Planting herbs too closely can lead to competition for resources, stunted growth, increased susceptibility to diseases, and reduced air circulation. Follow recommended spacing guidelines for each herb to ensure optimal growth and avoid overcrowding issues.

3. Neglecting Soil Quality:

The quality of your soil profoundly impacts the health of your medicinal herbs. Neglecting soil quality by not conducting soil tests, ignoring the need for amendments, or using poor-quality soil can lead to nutrient deficiencies, drainage problems, and overall poor plant health. Prioritize soil preparation, incorporate organic matter, and adjust soil pH based on the specific requirements of your herbs.

4. Overwatering or Underwatering:

Watering mistakes are common in herb gardening. Overwatering can lead to root rot, fungal diseases, and poor nutrient absorption, while underwatering results in stressed and weakened plants.

Develop a watering schedule based on the specific needs of each herb, monitor soil moisture regularly, and adjust your watering practices to seasonal changes.

5. Ignoring Sunlight Requirements:

Medicinal herbs have varying sunlight preferences, ranging from full sun to partial shade. Ignoring the sunlight requirements of your herbs can impact their growth and medicinal potency. Ensure that each herb receives the appropriate amount of sunlight based on its specific needs. Consider the natural habitat of the herb and mimic those conditions as closely as possible in your garden.

6. Skipping Pest and Disease Monitoring:

Pests and diseases can quickly compromise the health of your herb garden if not addressed promptly. Skipping regular monitoring for pests and diseases may result in infestations that are challenging to control. Implement preventive measures such as companion planting, maintaining good garden hygiene, and using organic pest control methods. Regularly inspect your herbs for any signs of pests or diseases to catch and address issues early.

7. Poor Plant Selection:

Selecting the wrong plants for your growing conditions or not considering the local climate can lead to disappointment. Before purchasing herbs, assess your hardiness zone, soil type, and overall climate. Choose herbs that are well-suited to your specific conditions to ensure they thrive and provide optimal medicinal benefits.

8. Neglecting Pruning and Harvesting Practices:

Pruning and harvesting are essential for maintaining the health and productivity of your medicinal herbs. Neglecting these practices can lead to leggy growth, reduced potency, and increased vulnerability to diseases. Learn the proper techniques for pruning and harvesting each herb, and follow recommended guidelines to encourage bushier, more robust plants.

9. Forgetting Companion Planting Principles:

Companion planting involves strategically placing plants that benefit each other when grown together.

Forgetting companion planting principles may result in missed opportunities for improved nutrient absorption, pest control, and overall plant health. Research companion plants for your medicinal herbs and implement these beneficial pairings to create a harmonious and supportive garden ecosystem.

10. Lack of Patience:

Impatience is a common mistake in herb gardening, particularly when waiting for plants to reach maturity or waiting for the first harvest. Rushing the growth process, skipping essential steps, or expecting instant results can lead to disappointment. Understand that growing medicinal herbs is a gradual and rewarding journey that requires patience and dedication.

Avoiding common mistakes is essential for a successful medicinal herb garden. By conducting thorough research, avoiding overcrowding, prioritizing soil quality, managing watering practices, considering sunlight requirements, monitoring for pests and diseases, making informed plant selections, practicing proper pruning and harvesting, embracing companion planting principles, and cultivating patience, you can create an environment that fosters the health, vitality, and medicinal potency of your herbs. Steer clear of these common pitfalls, and your medicinal herb garden is more likely to thrive and provide you with a bountiful harvest of potent and health-promoting plants.

Pest and Disease Management

Effective pest and disease management is crucial for maintaining a healthy and thriving medicinal herb garden. Pests and diseases can quickly undermine the well-being of your plants, leading to reduced growth, diminished medicinal potency, and even the loss of valuable herbs. Implementing proactive strategies and adopting sustainable practices can help prevent and address pest and disease issues in your garden. Here, we explore key considerations and tips for managing pests and diseases in your medicinal herb garden.

1. Identify and Monitor Pests:

Regularly inspect your medicinal herbs for signs of pests. Identify common pests such as aphids, mites, caterpillars, and beetles that may impact herb growth. Early detection is crucial for effective pest management. Look for chewed leaves, discoloration, or the presence of insects on the plants. Handpick pests when feasible, and use a magnifying glass if necessary to closely examine plant surfaces.

2. Encourage Beneficial Insects:

Natural predators play a significant role in pest management. Encourage beneficial insects such as ladybugs, lacewings, and predatory beetles in your garden. These insects feed on common pests, helping to maintain a balance in the ecosystem. Avoid using broad-spectrum insecticides that can harm beneficial insects along with pests. Planting companion plants that attract beneficial insects can further enhance natural pest control.

3. Practice Companion Planting:

Companion planting involves strategically placing plants that benefit each other when grown in close proximity. Certain herbs and flowers can repel or deter pests from your medicinal herbs. For example, planting basil, marigold, or nasturtium near susceptible herbs may help ward off pests. Research companion planting combinations that align with the specific needs of your medicinal herbs to create a pest-resistant garden.

4. Neem Oil and Horticultural Oils:

Neem oil and horticultural oils are effective organic options for managing pests. Neem oil disrupts the life cycle of insects, acting as an insect repellent and growth regulator. Horticultural oils suffocate pests by coating them, reducing their ability to breathe. These oils are safe for plants and beneficial insects when used according to instructions. Regular application can help prevent and control common pests.

5. Homemade Pest Repellents:

Create homemade pest repellents using common household ingredients. Garlic and chili pepper sprays can deter pests when applied to plants. A mixture of water, soap, and oil can be effective against soft-bodied insects. Experiment with natural repellents, and test them on a small portion of your herbs to ensure they don't cause harm before applying them more widely.

6. Beneficial Nematodes for Soil Health:

Beneficial nematodes are microscopic organisms that can help control soil-dwelling pests such as larvae of beetles, fleas, and moths. These nematodes actively seek out and infect pests, providing a natural and environmentally friendly pest management solution. Introduce beneficial nematodes to your soil to improve its overall health and reduce the population of harmful insects.

7. Implement Crop Rotation:

Crop rotation is an effective practice to manage soil-borne diseases and pests. Avoid planting the same family of herbs in the same location year after year. Rotating crops helps break the life cycle of pests and prevents the buildup of soil-borne pathogens. Plan your garden layout with crop rotation in mind to promote long-term soil health.

8. Proper Watering Practices:

Consistent and proper watering practices contribute to plant health and can help prevent certain diseases. Overhead watering, especially in the evening, can create a conducive environment for fungal diseases. Water at the base of plants in the morning to allow foliage to dry during the day. Avoid overwatering, as waterlogged soil can lead to root rot and other issues.

9. Cultural Practices for Disease Prevention:

Incorporate cultural practices that contribute to disease prevention. Prune plants to improve air circulation, remove diseased plant material promptly, and practice proper spacing to reduce humidity and minimize the risk of fungal infections. Sterilize gardening tools regularly to prevent the spread of diseases from one plant to another.

10. Use Disease-Resistant Varieties:

When selecting herbs for your garden, consider choosing disease-resistant varieties whenever possible. Disease-resistant plants have genetic traits that make them less susceptible to specific pathogens. Research and choose cultivars that are known for their resistance to common diseases in your region, providing an added layer of protection for your medicinal herbs.

11. Act Swiftly When Issues Arise:

Act swiftly if you notice signs of pests or diseases in your garden. Prompt intervention can prevent the escalation of the problem. Remove affected plant parts, isolate severely infected plants, and treat the issue using organic remedies or integrated pest management strategies. Regular monitoring and quick action contribute to the overall health of your medicinal herb garden.

12. Seek Professional Advice:

If pest or disease issues persist despite your efforts, don't hesitate to seek professional advice. Local agricultural extension offices, master gardeners, or experienced gardeners in your community may offer valuable insights and solutions tailored to your specific region and conditions. Professional guidance can help you address challenges effectively and make informed decisions for your medicinal herb garden.

Natural Pest Control Methods

Natural pest control methods are essential components of sustainable and eco-friendly gardening practices. When cultivating a medicinal herb garden, it's crucial to prioritize methods that not only protect your plants from pests but also maintain the overall health and integrity of the garden ecosystem. Here, we explore a variety of effective natural pest control methods that can be employed to keep your medicinal herbs thriving.

1. Beneficial Insects:

Harnessing the power of nature's own pest controllers is a cornerstone of natural pest control. Introduce or encourage beneficial insects in your garden, such as ladybugs, lacewings, predatory beetles, and parasitic wasps. These insects prey on common garden pests like aphids, caterpillars, and mites, helping to maintain a balanced and healthy ecosystem.

2. Neem Oil:

Neem oil, derived from the neem tree's seeds, is a potent natural insecticide and fungicide. It disrupts the life cycle of insects, acting as a repellent, growth regulator, and feeding deterrent. Neem oil is effective against a wide range of pests, including aphids, whiteflies, and spider mites. Regular application can help prevent infestations and protect your medicinal herbs without harming beneficial insects.

3. Homemade Insecticidal Soap:

Create your own insecticidal soap by combining water, liquid dish soap, and vegetable oil. This solution effectively controls soft-bodied pests like aphids, spider mites, and whiteflies. Apply the homemade insecticidal soap directly to the affected plants, ensuring thorough coverage. This method is a gentle yet powerful way to manage pests without resorting to chemical-based solutions.

4. Garlic Spray:

Garlic is known for its natural insect-repelling properties. Make a garlic spray by blending garlic cloves with water and straining the mixture. Dilute the solution and spray it on your medicinal herbs to deter pests. Garlic spray is particularly effective against aphids, caterpillars, and other soft-bodied insects. Regular applications can help protect your herbs while maintaining a chemical-free environment.

5. Companion Planting:

Companion planting involves strategically placing plants that benefit each other when grown in close proximity. Certain herbs and flowers can act as natural repellents against pests. For example, planting basil alongside tomatoes can help protect tomatoes from certain pests. Research companion planting combinations that align with the specific needs of your medicinal herbs to create a harmonious and pest-resistant garden.

6. Diatomaceous Earth:

Diatomaceous earth is a fine powder made from the fossilized remains of diatoms. It acts as a natural insecticide by dehydrating and damaging the exoskeletons of pests. Sprinkle diatomaceous earth around the base of your medicinal herbs to create a barrier against crawling insects. While harmless to humans and pets, diatomaceous earth is effective against pests like slugs, snails, and ants.

7. Hot Pepper Spray:

Hot pepper spray is an excellent natural deterrent for chewing insects and mammals. Create a homemade spray by blending hot peppers with water and a bit of dish soap. Strain the mixture and spray it on your herbs to discourage pests from feeding. This method is particularly useful against deer, rabbits, and certain insect pests.

8. Essential Oils:

Essential oils such as peppermint, lavender, and tea tree oil have potent insect-repelling properties. Dilute these oils in water and spray the solution on your medicinal herbs to deter pests. Essential oils not only protect against insects but also add aromatic qualities to your garden. Be mindful of the concentration, as excessive use may harm beneficial insects.

9. Beer Traps for Slugs and Snails:

Slugs and snails can be problematic in gardens, especially in damp conditions. Set up beer traps by burying containers with beer at soil level. Slugs and snails are attracted to the beer, fall in, and drown. Empty the traps regularly to keep them effective. Beer traps provide a simple and non-toxic way to control these common garden pests.

10. Planting Resistant Varieties:

Selecting herb varieties that are naturally resistant to common pests is a proactive approach to pest control. Choose cultivars that have built-in resistance to specific insects or diseases prevalent in your region. Resistant varieties often require less intervention, allowing you to maintain a more hands-off and sustainable gardening approach

11. Horticultural Oils:

Horticultural oils, such as neem oil and mineral oil, are effective natural pesticides that work by smothering and suffocating insects. These oils are particularly useful against soft-bodied pests like aphids, scales, and mites. Ensure proper dilution and application, and use horticultural oils as part of an integrated pest management strategy.

12. Crop Rotation:

Implementing a crop rotation plan is a natural way to disrupt the life cycle of pests and reduce the risk of soil-borne diseases. Avoid planting herbs from the same family in the same location year after year. Rotate crops to different areas of your garden, promoting a healthier soil environment and minimizing pest **buildup.**

13. Yellow Sticky Traps:

Yellow sticky traps are an effective method for monitoring and controlling flying insect pests. These traps are coated with a sticky substance that captures flying insects when they come in contact. Hang yellow sticky traps around your medicinal herb garden to control pests like whiteflies, fungus gnats, and aphids. Regularly replace the traps to maintain their efficacy.

14. Pruning and Removing Infected Plant Parts:

Pruning and promptly removing infected or infested plant parts can help contain the spread of diseases and pests. Regularly inspect your medicinal herbs for signs of infection or damage, and trim affected areas to prevent the issue from spreading. Proper sanitation practices contribute to the overall health of your garden.

15. Sticky Barriers for Crawling Insects:

Sticky barriers, such as Tanglefoot or other sticky substances, can be applied around the base of plants to create a physical barrier against crawling insects. These barriers are effective against ants, caterpillars, and other pests that travel along plant stems. Regularly check and replenish sticky barriers as needed.

Identifying Common Diseases

Identifying and understanding common diseases affecting medicinal herbs is crucial for maintaining a healthy and productive garden.

Recognizing the signs and symptoms of diseases early on allows for timely intervention and effective management strategies. Here, we explore some of the most prevalent diseases that can impact medicinal herbs, along with key characteristics to help you identify and address them in your garden.

1. Powdery Mildew:

> **Characteristics:**

Powdery mildew is a common fungal disease characterized by the presence of a white, powdery substance on the surfaces of leaves, stems, and sometimes flowers. It often thrives in warm and dry conditions.

> **Affected Herbs:**

Powdery mildew can affect a wide range of herbs, including mint, basil, oregano, and rosemary.

> **Management Strategies:**

Increase air circulation by spacing plants adequately.

Water at the base of plants to keep foliage dry.

Apply fungicidal sprays or organic remedies like neem oil.

2. Downy Mildew:

> **Characteristics:**

Downy mildew is another fungal disease, but it appears as yellow or brownish patches on the upper surface of leaves. The underside of affected leaves may exhibit a downy, purplish growth.

> **Affected Herbs:**

Downy mildew can impact herbs like basil, sage, and mint.

> **Management Strategies:**

Provide proper spacing to improve air circulation.

Avoid overhead watering.

Apply copper-based fungicides or organic alternatives.

3. Fusarium Wilt:

> **Characteristics:**

Fusarium wilt is a soil-borne disease caused by the Fusarium fungus. It leads to wilting, yellowing, and stunting of plants. Vascular tissues may exhibit discoloration.

> **Affected Herbs:**

Basil is particularly susceptible to Fusarium wilt.

> **Management Strategies:**

Plant resistant varieties.

Practice crop rotation.

Avoid overwatering and improve soil drainage.

4. Root Rot:

> **Characteristics:**

Root rot is caused by various fungi, including Phytophthora and Rhizoctonia. It results in the decay of roots, leading to wilting, yellowing, and collapse of the entire plant.

> **Affected Herbs:**

Herbs like thyme and lavender may be susceptible to root rot.

> **Management Strategies:**

Ensure well-draining soil.

Avoid overwatering and provide proper aeration.

Apply fungicides containing beneficial microorganisms.

5. Rust:

> ### Characteristics:

Rust diseases manifest as orange or reddish-brown pustules on the undersides of leaves. These pustules release spores, contributing to the spread of the disease.

> ### Affected Herbs:

Mint and oregano can be prone to rust.

> ### Management Strategies:

Remove infected plant material promptly.

Apply sulfur-based fungicides.

Maintain good air circulation.

6. Bacterial Leaf Spot:

> ### Characteristics:

Bacterial leaf spot causes dark, water-soaked lesions on leaves, which may have a yellow halo. It is caused by bacteria and spreads through water and soil.

> ### Affected Herbs:

Basil and parsley are susceptible to bacterial leaf spot.

> ### Management Strategies:

Water at the base to avoid splashing.

Remove infected leaves.

Apply copper-based sprays.

7. Gray Mold (Botrytis):

> **Characteristics:**

Gray mold, caused by the Botrytis fungus, leads to fuzzy gray or brown growth on leaves, stems, and flowers. It thrives in cool and humid conditions.

> **Affected Herbs:**

Botrytis can affect a variety of herbs, including thyme and sage.

> **Management Strategies:**

Ensure good air circulation.

Remove and dispose of infected plant material.

Apply fungicides, especially during cool and damp weather.

8. Aphid Infestations:

> **Characteristics:**

While not a disease, aphids are common pests that can cause significant damage. These small, soft-bodied insects cluster on plant stems and leaves, sucking sap and causing leaf curling.

> **Affected Herbs:**

Aphids can infest various herbs, including mint, rosemary, and basil.

> **Management Strategies:**

Introduce beneficial insects like ladybugs.

Use a strong stream of water to dislodge aphids.

Apply neem oil or insecticidal soaps.

9. Spider Mites:

> **Characteristics:**

Spider mites are tiny arachnids that feed on plant sap, causing stippling, discoloration, and webbing on the undersides of leaves.

Affected Herbs:

Mint and rosemary can be susceptible to spider mite infestations.

> **Management Strategies:**

Increase humidity to deter mites.

Apply insecticidal soaps or neem oil.

Introduce predatory mites or insects.

10. Whiteflies:

> **Characteristics:**

Whiteflies are small, winged insects that cluster on the undersides of leaves. They suck sap and excrete honeydew, leading to sooty mold growth.

> **Affected Herbs:**

Basil and thyme are among the herbs that whiteflies may infest.

> **Management Strategies:**

Use yellow sticky traps to monitor and trap whiteflies.

Apply insecticidal soaps or neem oil.

Introduce natural predators like parasitic wasps.

11. Cucumber Mosaic Virus (CMV):

> **Characteristics:**

CMV causes mosaic patterns on leaves, stunting, and yellowing. It is transmitted by aphids and can affect a wide range of plants, including herbs.

> **Affected Herbs:**

Mint and oregano may be susceptible to Cucumber Mosaic Virus.

> **Management Strategies:**

Control aphid populations.

Remove and destroy infected plants.

Plant virus-resistant herb varieties.

12. Septoria Leaf Spot:

> **Characteristics:**

Septoria leaf spot appears as small, dark spots with a lighter center on leaves. It is caused by a fungus and can lead to defoliation.

> **Affected Herbs:**

Basil is commonly affected by Septoria leaf spot.

> **Management Strategies:**

Provide adequate spacing for air circulation.

Water at the base to avoid leaf wetting.

Apply copper-based fungicides.

13. Tomato Spotted Wilt Virus (TSWV):

> ➢ **Characteristics:**

TSWV causes yellowing, wilting, and bronzing of leaves. It is transmitted by thrips, tiny insects that feed on plant juices.

> ➢ **Affected Herbs:**

Thyme and parsley may be susceptible to Tomato Spotted Wilt Virus.

> ➢ **Management Strategies:**

Control thrips populations.

Remove and destroy infected plants.

Plant virus-resistant varieties.

14. Crown Gall:

> ➢ **Characteristics:**

Crown gall is caused by a bacterium and leads to the development of tumor-like growths on roots and stems.

> ➢ **Affected Herbs:**

Various herbs can be impacted by crown gall.

> ➢ **Management Strategies:**

Remove and destroy infected plants.

Practice proper sanitation to prevent bacterial spread.

Plant disease-free herb material.

15. Verticillium Wilt:

> **Characteristics:**

Verticillium wilt causes wilting, yellowing, and vascular discoloration. It is caused by soil-borne fungi and can persist in the soil for years.

> **Affected Herbs:**

Herbs like lavender and rosemary may be susceptible to Verticillium wilt.

> **Management Strategies:**

Plant resistant varieties.

Practice crop rotation.

Provide optimal soil drainage.

Pruning and Training Techniques

Pruning and training techniques are essential practices for maintaining the health, shape, and productivity of medicinal herb plants. These horticultural methods not only help control the size and structure of the plants but also contribute to improved air circulation, sunlight penetration, and overall vigor. Here, we explore various pruning and training techniques that can be applied to medicinal herbs to enhance their growth and maximize their medicinal potency.

1. Pinching:

Pinching involves the removal of the terminal bud or shoot tip, usually done with fingers or pruning shears. This technique stimulates lateral branching, resulting in a bushier and more compact plant. Pinching is commonly used for herbs like basil, oregano, and mint. By pinching regularly, you encourage the development of side shoots, leading to increased foliage and potential medicinal compounds.

2. Deadheading:

Deadheading is the removal of spent or faded flowers from a plant. For medicinal herbs that produce flowers, such as chamomile or lavender, deadheading redirects the plant's energy from seed production to vegetative growth. This encourages the continuous production of new flowers and prolongs the overall flowering period. Deadheading also enhances the appearance of the plant and prevents self-seeding.

3. Thinning:

Thinning involves the selective removal of entire branches or stems to reduce plant density. This technique is particularly useful for herbs like rosemary or sage, which can become dense and woody over time. Thinning helps improve air circulation, reduce disease susceptibility, and promote the penetration of sunlight into the plant's interior. It also prevents overcrowding and enhances the overall aesthetic appeal of the herb.

4. Crown Pruning:

Crown pruning focuses on removing the upper portion or crown of the plant. This technique is beneficial for herbs like thyme or lavender, especially when they exhibit excessive woody growth in the center. Crown pruning rejuvenates the plant, encourages new growth from the base, and prevents the development of a leggy or unproductive center. It is essential to use sharp pruning tools for clean cuts to minimize stress on the plant.

5. Rejuvenation Pruning:

Rejuvenation pruning involves cutting back the entire plant to stimulate new and vigorous growth. This technique is suitable for perennial herbs that may become woody or leggy over time, such as sage or oregano. Rejuvenation pruning is typically done in late winter or early spring before the growing season begins. While the initial cut may seem drastic, the plant responds by producing fresh shoots and foliage.

6. Espalier:

Espalier is a training technique that involves growing plants in a flat, two-dimensional form against a support structure, such as a trellis or wall. While often associated with fruit trees, this method can be applied to certain climbing or vining herbs like thyme or lemon balm. Espaliering herbs not only saves space but also facilitates better sunlight exposure and air circulation, leading to healthier growth.

7. Topiary:

Topiary involves shaping and pruning plants into ornamental and geometric forms. While traditionally associated with ornamental plants, certain herbs like rosemary or lavender can be shaped into topiary designs. Topiary not only adds an aesthetic element to the garden but also helps control the size and form of the herbs. Regular shaping and trimming maintain the desired topiary structure.

8. Training on Supports:

Some medicinal herbs, such as climbing or vining varieties, benefit from being trained onto supports. This could include trellises, stakes, or other structures that guide the plant's growth. Herbs like hops or climbing roses can be trained vertically, utilizing supports to maximize sunlight exposure and optimize space. Training also prevents sprawling growth and makes harvesting easier.

9. Pruning for Concentrated Essential Oils:

For herbs valued for their essential oils, such as lavender or basil, specific pruning techniques can enhance oil concentration. Prune these herbs during the morning when essential oil levels are highest, and avoid pruning during flowering to prevent disruption of oil production. Additionally, removing flowers after they bloom redirects the plant's energy toward oil synthesis, resulting in more potent aromatic compounds.

10. Lateral Pruning:

Lateral pruning focuses on removing side shoots or lateral branches to shape the plant and encourage upward growth. This technique is particularly useful for herbs like mint or oregano. Lateral pruning helps maintain a more compact and controlled plant size, prevents sprawling, and enhances the overall appearance of the herb.

11. Cut-and-Come-Again Harvesting:

While not traditional pruning, the cut-and-come-again harvesting approach involves regularly harvesting the outer leaves or stems of herbs without removing the entire plant. This method is suitable for continuous harvest herbs like parsley or cilantro. By harvesting selectively, you encourage the growth of new shoots, ensuring a continuous supply of fresh leaves throughout the growing season.

12. Pollarding:

Pollarding is a severe pruning technique that involves cutting back the upper branches of a tree or shrub to control its size and shape. While not commonly applied to medicinal herbs, certain perennial varieties with woody growth, like rosemary, can benefit from controlled pollarding to rejuvenate the plant and encourage denser foliage.

13. Controlling Spread:

For herbs that tend to spread aggressively, such as mint or lemon balm, controlling their growth is essential. Regularly prune or trim the outer edges of the plant to prevent it from invading neighboring areas. Using physical barriers like buried containers or edging can also help contain the spread of invasive herbs.

14. Sucker Removal:

Suckers are shoots that emerge from the base of the plant, often near the soil level. Removing suckers is crucial for maintaining the desired form and preventing the plant from becoming unruly. This technique is commonly applied to herbs like thyme or sage. Regularly inspect the base of the plant and prune away any unwanted suckers.

15. Winter Pruning:

Winter pruning is performed during the dormant season and is particularly beneficial for deciduous herbs like rosemary or lavender. This technique involves removing dead or damaged wood, shaping the plant, and thinning out crowded growth. Winter pruning sets the stage for vigorous spring growth and ensures a healthy and well-structured plant.

Promoting Healthy Growth

Promoting healthy growth in medicinal herbs is a fundamental aspect of successful cultivation, ensuring robust plants with optimal medicinal potency. To achieve this, gardeners must implement a holistic approach that addresses various factors, including soil quality, watering practices, sunlight exposure, nutrient management, and pest control. Here, we explore key strategies for fostering the healthy growth of medicinal herbs, contributing to a flourishing and productive garden.

1. Soil Quality and Preparation:

Healthy growth begins with the soil. Ensure your medicinal herbs are planted in well-draining, nutrient-rich soil. Conduct a soil test to assess pH levels and nutrient content, and amend the soil accordingly. Incorporate organic matter such as compost or well-rotted manure to enhance soil structure and fertility. Proper soil preparation creates an optimal foundation for robust root development and nutrient absorption.

2. Correct Plant Spacing:

Proper plant spacing is essential for preventing overcrowding, ensuring adequate air circulation, and minimizing competition for nutrients. Research the specific spacing requirements for each herb in your garden and adhere to these guidelines during planting. Well-spaced plants not only receive sufficient sunlight but also experience reduced risks of diseases due to improved airflow.

3. Adequate Sunlight Exposure:

Most medicinal herbs thrive in full sunlight, receiving at least 6-8 hours of direct sunlight daily. Adequate sunlight exposure promotes photosynthesis, essential for the production of sugars and plant growth. Ensure that your garden is situated in a location that receives ample sunlight, and position herbs according to their sunlight preferences. Consider the natural habitat of each herb when planning your garden layout.

4. Proper Watering Practices:

Consistent and appropriate watering is crucial for promoting healthy growth. Overwatering can lead to root rot and other fungal diseases, while underwatering stresses plants and hampers growth. Develop a watering schedule based on the specific needs of each herb, considering factors such as soil type, climate, and individual water requirements. Water at the base of plants to prevent wet foliage, especially in the evening, which can contribute to fungal issues.

5. Mulching for Moisture Retention:

Mulching is an effective technique for retaining soil moisture, regulating temperature, and suppressing weeds. Apply a layer of organic mulch around the base of medicinal herbs to conserve moisture, reduce evaporation, and create a more stable soil environment. Mulching also contributes to weed control, preventing unwanted competition for nutrients and water.

6. Balanced Nutrition:

Providing balanced nutrition is essential for supporting healthy growth and maximizing medicinal potency. Fertilize your medicinal herbs with a well-balanced, organic fertilizer, taking into account their specific nutrient requirements. Consider applying compost or organic amendments periodically to enrich the soil with essential micronutrients. Avoid over-fertilizing, as excessive nutrients can lead to imbalances and negatively impact plant health.

7. Pruning and Deadheading:

Regular pruning and deadheading are key practices for promoting healthy growth in medicinal herbs. Pruning helps shape the plant, improve air circulation, and stimulate lateral branching. Deadheading redirects the plant's energy toward new growth, prolongs flowering, and enhances overall aesthetics. Tailor your pruning approach to the specific needs of each herb, considering their growth habits and life cycles.

8. Integrated Pest Management (IPM):

Implementing Integrated Pest Management is crucial for preventing and managing pest issues that can compromise plant health. Regularly inspect your herbs for signs of pests and diseases, and intervene promptly when necessary. Utilize natural predators, companion planting, and organic pest control methods to minimize the use of chemical pesticides. Maintaining a healthy ecosystem in your garden helps control pest populations without harming beneficial insects.

9. Companion Planting:

Companion planting involves strategically placing plants that benefit each other when grown together. Incorporate companion plants that deter pests, attract beneficial insects, or provide natural protection to your medicinal herbs. For example, planting basil alongside tomatoes can help deter certain pests. Companion planting contributes to a balanced and resilient garden ecosystem.

10. Regular Monitoring and Observation:

Regular monitoring and observation are essential for detecting early signs of stress, diseases, or pest infestations. Establish a routine for inspecting your medicinal herbs, checking for changes in foliage color, growth patterns, or any abnormal symptoms. Swift intervention based on keen observation contributes to the overall health and longevity of your herbal garden.

11. Propagation and Renewal:

Regularly propagate and renew your herbs to maintain vigorous growth. Propagation methods such as division, cuttings, or seed sowing help refresh plant stock, rejuvenate older specimens, and ensure a continuous supply of healthy herbs. Propagate herbs during the appropriate season, taking into account their specific growth habits and reproductive cycles.

12. Adequate Support for Tall or Climbing Herbs:

Provide adequate support for tall or climbing herbs to prevent them from bending or breaking under their weight. Use stakes, cages, or trellises to support plants like tomatoes, sage, or climbing varieties. Proper support ensures that stems remain upright, reducing the risk of damage and promoting healthy growth.

13. Seasonal Care:

Adjust your care practices based on the seasons. In colder climates, protect herbs from frost, and in hot climates, provide shade during the hottest part of the day. Seasonal care also includes adapting watering schedules, adjusting fertilization, and monitoring for seasonal pests and diseases.

14. Selecting Resilient Varieties:

When choosing herbs for your garden, consider selecting varieties known for their resilience and adaptability to your specific climate and growing conditions. Resilient varieties are more likely to withstand environmental stressors, diseases, and pests, promoting overall plant health and longevity.

15. Soil Aeration:

Ensure proper soil aeration to facilitate root respiration and nutrient absorption. Compacted or waterlogged soil can hinder root development and lead to issues such as root rot. Regularly aerate the soil by loosening it with a fork or other suitable tools, especially in heavy clay soils.

Shaping and Controlling Size

Shaping and controlling the size of medicinal herbs is a vital aspect of herb cultivation that contributes to the overall health, aesthetics, and functionality of the garden. Proper shaping enhances the plant's form, promotes optimal sunlight exposure, improves air circulation, and facilitates easier harvesting. Additionally, controlling size is essential for preventing overcrowding, which can lead to increased vulnerability to pests and diseases. Here, we explore various techniques for shaping and controlling the size of medicinal herbs, ensuring a well-maintained and productive garden.

1. Pruning for Form:

Pruning is a fundamental technique for shaping medicinal herbs and maintaining an attractive form. Depending on the growth habit of each herb, pruning can involve the removal of excessive foliage, dead or damaged branches, or the shaping of the overall structure.

For example, herbs like basil and mint benefit from regular pinching to encourage bushier growth, while rosemary or lavender may require selective pruning to maintain a compact and tidy appearance.

2. Selective Removal of Overgrown Stems:

Overgrown or leggy stems can detract from the overall aesthetics of medicinal herbs and compromise their health. Selective removal of these stems helps maintain a balanced and visually pleasing plant. Use sharp pruning shears to cut back overgrown stems to a junction with healthy foliage. This encourages new growth from the base and prevents the plant from becoming too top-heavy.

3. Controlling Spread:

Certain medicinal herbs, such as mint and lemon balm, are known for their vigorous spreading habits. To prevent these herbs from taking over the garden, install physical barriers like buried containers or edging to control their lateral growth. Regularly prune the outer edges of the plant to contain its spread and redirect energy to the central growth.

4. Espalier or Trellising:

Espalier and trellising techniques are effective for herbs that exhibit a vining or climbing growth habit. Train the herb to grow along a flat, two-dimensional surface, such as a trellis or wall. This not only controls the plant's size but also maximizes sunlight exposure and facilitates easier harvesting. Espalier is particularly suitable for herbs like thyme or climbing varieties of rosemary.

5. Size-Appropriate Containers:

When cultivating medicinal herbs in containers, selecting appropriately sized pots is crucial for controlling their size. Herbs like sage or basil can become root-bound if confined to small containers, hindering their growth and overall health. Choose containers with sufficient depth and width to accommodate the specific root structure of each herb, allowing for proper development.

6. Root Pruning during Transplanting:

During transplanting, especially when moving herbs from containers to the ground or larger pots, consider root pruning. Gently trim the outer edges of the root ball before replanting to encourage the development of new, more compact roots. Root pruning prevents the herb from becoming root-bound and promotes healthier growth in its new location.

7. Crown Pruning for Woody Herbs:

For woody herbs like rosemary or lavender, crown pruning is an effective technique for controlling size and rejuvenating the plant. Remove the upper portion or crown of the plant to stimulate new growth from the base. This helps prevent the development of a leggy or woody center, maintaining a more compact and lush appearance.

8. Seasonal Pruning:

Adjust your pruning practices according to the seasons to accommodate the growth cycles of medicinal herbs. Perform more extensive pruning, if needed, during the dormant season or early spring to shape the plant before the onset of active growth. Seasonal pruning helps maintain a balanced and well-structured plant throughout the year.

9. Containment in Raised Beds:

Growing medicinal herbs in raised beds offers the advantage of better soil drainage and allows for more controlled growth. Build raised beds with suitable dimensions for each herb, preventing them from spreading excessively. Additionally, raised beds provide easy access for maintenance and harvesting.

10. Bonsai Techniques for Compact Growth:

Bonsai techniques can be applied to certain herbs to achieve compact and controlled growth. While not traditional for all herbs, experimenting with bonsai methods, such as root pruning and selective trimming, can result in smaller, aesthetically pleasing specimens. Research specific bonsai techniques applicable to the herb species you are cultivating.

11. Cut-and-Come-Again Harvesting:

Incorporate cut-and-come-again harvesting practices to control size and encourage continuous growth. Rather than harvesting the entire plant at once, selectively harvest mature leaves or stems while leaving the plant's central growth intact. This approach allows the herb to continuously produce new foliage, extending the harvesting period and maintaining an overall compact size.

12. Avoiding Overcrowding:

Prevent overcrowding by adhering to recommended plant spacing guidelines. Overcrowded plants compete for resources, leading to decreased air circulation, increased susceptibility to diseases, and stunted growth. Proper spacing ensures each herb has sufficient room to grow and thrive.

13. Monitoring and Adjusting Growth:

Regularly monitor the growth of medicinal herbs and adjust cultivation practices accordingly. If a particular herb is showing signs of overgrowth or spreading too aggressively, intervene with targeted pruning or other size-controlling measures. Adjustments may be necessary based on seasonal variations, environmental conditions, or changes in the garden ecosystem.

14. Height Control for Indoor Cultivation:

For indoor cultivation of medicinal herbs, controlling height is crucial to prevent plants from outgrowing their designated space. Employ techniques like topping or bending to manage height and promote bushier growth. Additionally, adjust light intensity and duration to influence growth patterns and prevent elongation.

15. Avoiding Excessive Fertilization:

While providing adequate nutrition is essential for healthy growth, excessive fertilization can lead to overly vigorous growth and larger-than-desired plants. Follow recommended fertilization schedules, and avoid overfeeding herbs. Balanced nutrition supports optimal growth without promoting excessive size.

Shaping and controlling the size of medicinal herbs are integral components of successful herb cultivation. By incorporating pruning techniques, utilizing appropriate containers, employing trellising or espalier methods, practicing root pruning during transplanting, and adopting other size-controlling measures, gardeners can create a well-balanced and visually appealing herb garden. These strategies not only contribute to the overall health and longevity of medicinal herbs but also enhance the garden's functionality and aesthetic appeal.

Harvesting Guidelines

Harvesting medicinal herbs is a crucial step in the cultivation process, marking the culmination of efforts invested in nurturing plants to their full potential.

The timing, methods, and considerations during harvesting significantly impact the quality and potency of the herbs. Whether you're cultivating herbs for culinary, medicinal, or aromatic purposes, following proper harvesting guidelines ensures a bountiful and potent yield while promoting the long-term health of the plants. Here are essential guidelines to consider when harvesting medicinal herbs:

1. Timing is Critical:

Harvesting herbs at the right time is essential to maximize their medicinal potency and flavor. Different herbs have varying peak harvesting times, often coinciding with specific stages of their growth cycles. Harvesting is typically done just before or during the flowering stage when essential oil concentrations are at their highest. However, for herbs prized for their leaves, like basil or mint, harvesting before flowering ensures optimal flavor and aroma.

2. Morning Harvests for Best Quality:

Early morning is generally the best time for harvesting medicinal herbs. At this time, the essential oil content is highest, and the plants are less stressed by the heat of the day. Harvesting in the morning preserves the herb's flavor, aroma, and medicinal compounds. If morning harvesting is not feasible, late afternoon is the second-best option.

3. Consider the Growth Stage:

Each herb has a specific growth stage when it is most beneficial to harvest. For leafy herbs like parsley or cilantro, the leaves are typically harvested before the plant flowers. For herbs valued for their flowers, such as chamomile or lavender, harvesting during full bloom is ideal. Understanding the growth habits of each herb guides you in selecting the right harvesting time.

4. Use Clean and Sharp Tools:

Always use clean and sharp tools when harvesting herbs. Clean tools reduce the risk of transmitting diseases between plants, while sharp tools make clean cuts, minimizing stress on the plants. Pruning shears, scissors, or a sharp knife are suitable for harvesting, depending on the size and density of the plant.

5. Harvesting Frequency:

Incorporate a regular harvesting schedule to encourage continuous growth and maintain plant vitality. For many herbs, such as basil or oregano, frequent harvesting promotes branching and results in a bushier, more productive plant. However, avoid overharvesting, as it may stress the plant and compromise its overall health.

6. Harvesting Whole Plants vs. Selective Harvesting:

The decision to harvest the entire plant or selectively harvest specific parts depends on the herb and its growth habits. For perennial herbs like thyme or rosemary, selective harvesting of stems or leaves allows the plant to continue producing over an extended period. Annual herbs like basil or cilantro may be harvested more comprehensively. Consider the plant's growth habits and your intended use when deciding on the harvesting approach.

7. Proper Techniques for Leafy Herbs:

Leafy herbs such as basil, mint, or cilantro require specific harvesting techniques to encourage continual growth. Pinch or cut stems just above a set of leaves to promote branching and a fuller appearance. Avoid removing more than one-third of the plant at a time to prevent stress and allow for quick recovery.

8. Harvesting Flowers:

For herbs valued for their flowers, such as chamomile or calendula, harvest when the blooms are fully open. Gently cut the flowers, leaving some stem attached. Avoid harvesting flowers that show signs of discoloration or wilting, as these may not have the highest concentration of essential oils.

9. Harvesting Roots:

For herbs with medicinal roots, such as echinacea or valerian, harvesting is typically done in the fall when the energy of the plant has moved downward. Use a garden fork or spade to carefully unearth the roots, ensuring minimal damage. Wash and clean the roots thoroughly before drying or processing.

10. Drying Techniques:

After harvesting, proper drying techniques are essential to preserve the quality of medicinal herbs. Arrange leaves, flowers, or roots in a single layer on drying racks, screens, or in bundles tied loosely with twine. Ensure good air circulation to prevent mold or mildew. Dry herbs in a dark, well-ventilated area away from direct sunlight. Roots may take longer to dry, and proper ventilation is crucial to prevent moisture buildup.

11. Storage Considerations:

Once dried, store herbs in airtight containers, away from heat, light, and moisture. Glass jars or opaque containers help maintain the herbs' quality by protecting them from exposure to sunlight. Label containers with the herb's name and harvest date for easy identification. Proper storage preserves the potency and flavor of medicinal herbs for an extended period.

12. Consider Environmental Factors:

Be mindful of environmental factors when harvesting herbs. Avoid harvesting after heavy rainfall or during extremely humid conditions, as excess moisture can impact the quality of the herbs. Similarly, refrain from harvesting during times of extreme heat, as herbs may be stressed and more susceptible to wilting.

13. Sustainable Harvesting Practices:

Adopt sustainable harvesting practices to ensure the long-term viability of medicinal herbs. Avoid harvesting more than a third of the plant population in a given area. Consider implementing rotational harvesting, allowing certain areas to recover while others are harvested. This approach promotes ecological balance and ensures the continued health of the herb population.

14. Harvesting for Seed Saving:

When harvesting herbs for seed saving, allow the plants to reach full maturity before collecting seeds. Harvest seeds when they are fully developed and have turned brown or are easily separated from the plant. Place harvested seeds in a dry, well-ventilated area to complete the drying process before storing them in airtight containers.

15. Research Individual Herbs:

Lastly, individual herbs may have specific considerations for harvesting. Some herbs may require special attention to certain parts, growth habits, or timing. Research the specific requirements of each herb in your garden to tailor your harvesting practices accordingly.

Harvesting medicinal herbs is a skill that improves with experience and understanding of each herb's unique characteristics. By considering factors such as timing, cleanliness, tools, frequency, and drying techniques, you can optimize the quality and quantity of your herbal harvest.

Following these guidelines ensures a sustainable and rewarding practice, providing you with a continuous supply of potent and flavorful herbs from your garden.

Optimal Harvest Times

Determining the optimal harvest time is a crucial aspect of cultivating medicinal herbs, as it directly influences the concentration of essential oils, flavors, and therapeutic compounds within the plants. The ideal harvesting period varies among different herbs, and factors such as growth stage, environmental conditions, and intended use play significant roles. Here, we explore the key considerations for determining optimal harvest times to maximize the potency and quality of medicinal herbs.

1. Growth Stage:

Understanding the growth stages of medicinal herbs is fundamental to selecting the optimal harvest time. Herbs go through distinct phases, including vegetative growth, flowering, and seed setting. For leafy herbs like basil or mint, harvesting during the vegetative stage, before flowering, generally results in the highest essential oil content and flavor. Conversely, herbs valued for their flowers, such as chamomile or lavender, are typically harvested during full bloom for maximum potency.

2. Flowering Stage for Floral Herbs:

Herbs with prominent flowers often reach their peak potency during the flowering stage. Chamomile, calendula, and lavender are examples where harvesting during full bloom ensures the highest concentration of aromatic compounds and therapeutic benefits. Flowers are generally harvested when they are fully open, displaying vibrant colors and fragrances.

3. Leaf Harvesting Before Flowering:

For herbs grown for their leaves, such as basil, oregano, or cilantro, the optimal harvest time is typically before the plants enter the flowering stage. Harvesting before flowering ensures that the plant's energy is directed towards producing flavorful leaves rather than seeds. This stage often results in the highest concentration of essential oils and a more robust flavor profile.

4. Early Morning Harvests:

Harvesting medicinal herbs early in the morning, when the dew has dried but before the heat of the day, is generally recommended.

At this time, the essential oil content is often at its peak. Morning harvests help preserve the plant's vitality and prevent wilting, leading to better quality herbs with higher concentrations of active compounds.

5. Seasonal Considerations:

Seasonal variations also impact the optimal harvest time for medicinal herbs. In colder climates, the growing season may be shorter, requiring careful timing to capture the peak potency of the herbs. In warmer regions, where plants may continue to thrive for an extended period, repeated harvesting throughout the season may be possible.

6. Avoiding Stressful Conditions:

Harvesting herbs during stressful conditions, such as extreme heat or drought, can affect their quality. Plants under stress may redirect their resources away from essential oil production, leading to diminished potency. Aim to harvest during periods of moderate temperature and adequate soil moisture to ensure optimal conditions for the plants.

7. Consideration of Individual Herbs:

Different herbs have distinct growth habits and optimal harvest times. Conduct thorough research on each herb in your garden to understand its specific requirements. For example, harvesting basil just before it starts to flower ensures a more potent flavor, while harvesting rosemary during the flowering stage may yield higher concentrations of essential oils.

8. Monitoring Plant Appearance:

Observing the physical appearance of the plant is a practical way to gauge its readiness for harvest. Look for signs such as vibrant color, well-developed leaves, and full blooms, depending on the plant type. Additionally, some herbs may exhibit changes in leaf texture or aroma, indicating the optimal time for harvest.

9. Testing Essential Oil Content:

For those cultivating medicinal herbs for essential oil extraction, testing the oil content can provide valuable insights into the optimal harvest time. Essential oil content is often influenced by factors such as growth stage, time of day, and environmental conditions. Testing can be done using specialized equipment or by consulting with experts in herbal extraction.

10. Harvesting for Culinary Herbs:

When growing herbs for culinary purposes, the optimal harvest time is often determined by the plant part used. Leafy herbs like parsley or cilantro are typically harvested before flowering for the best flavor. For culinary herbs valued for their seeds, such as dill or coriander, harvesting occurs when the seeds are fully developed and easy to collect.

11. Harvesting Medicinal Roots:

Herbs with medicinal roots, like echinacea or valerian, are typically harvested in the fall when the plant's energy has moved downward. This ensures that the roots have accumulated the maximum concentration of beneficial compounds. Use caution during root harvesting to minimize damage and preserve the plant's overall health.

12. Regular Monitoring and Adjustment:

Continuous monitoring of your herbal garden is essential to adjust harvesting times based on the changing needs of the plants. Regular inspections allow you to identify signs of flowering, detect potential pest issues, and make timely decisions to optimize the harvest.

13. Environmental Factors:

Environmental factors, including sunlight, temperature, and humidity, influence the growth and potency of medicinal herbs. Harvesting during favorable weather conditions contributes to the overall quality of the herbs. Avoid harvesting during excessively hot or humid periods, as these conditions may impact the essential oil content and overall vitality of the plants.

14. Balancing Growth and Harvest:

Balancing the need for harvest with the plant's ongoing growth is crucial for maintaining a sustainable and productive garden. Frequent harvesting, when done judiciously, can encourage continual growth and increased yields. However, overharvesting may stress the plants, leading to diminished vitality and potential long-term harm.

15. Expert Consultation:

Seeking guidance from experienced herbalists, local horticulturists, or agricultural extension services can provide valuable insights into the optimal harvest times for specific medicinal herbs in your region.

Local knowledge, combined with hands-on experience, enhances your ability to make informed decisions regarding harvest timing.

Determining the optimal harvest time for medicinal herbs is a nuanced process that requires attention to various factors. By considering growth stages, flowering patterns, environmental conditions, and individual herb characteristics, you can enhance the potency and quality of your herbal harvest. Regular monitoring, expert consultation, and a deep understanding of each herb contribute to a successful and rewarding cultivation experience.

Drying and Storing Herbs

Drying and storing herbs effectively is a crucial step in preserving their potency, flavor, and aroma for future use. Whether cultivating medicinal herbs for health, culinary herbs for flavor, or aromatic herbs for sensory enjoyment, the proper drying and storage techniques ensure a longer shelf life and maintain the herbs' essential qualities. Here are essential guidelines for drying and storing herbs to maximize their benefits and enjoyment:

1. Timing of Harvest and Drying:

The timing of harvest significantly influences the quality of dried herbs. Harvest herbs when essential oil concentrations are at their peak, usually in the morning after dew has dried but before the heat of the day intensifies. This timing ensures optimal flavor and medicinal potency. Avoid harvesting during or after rainfall, as damp herbs are more prone to mold during the drying process.

2. Air Drying:

Air drying is one of the oldest and simplest methods for preserving herbs. Gather small bundles of herbs, tie them with twine, and hang them upside down in a cool, dark, and well-ventilated area. The bundles should not be too large to promote proper air circulation. This method is suitable for leafy herbs like basil, mint, or oregano.

3. Drying Rack or Screen:

Using a drying rack or screen is an effective alternative to hanging herbs. Place the herbs in a single layer on a rack or screen, allowing air to circulate around each leaf or flower. Ensure the drying location is well-ventilated and away from direct sunlight to prevent the degradation of essential oils.

4. Dehydrators:

Dehydrators offer a controlled environment for drying herbs, maintaining consistent temperature and air circulation. This method is particularly useful for large quantities of herbs or in areas with high humidity. Follow the dehydrator's instructions and set it to a low temperature to preserve the herbs' essential oils.

5. Microwave Drying:

While less common, the microwave can be used for quick herb drying. Place herbs between layers of paper towels and microwave in short intervals until the herbs are dry. This method is suitable for small batches, but be cautious not to overheat or burn the herbs.

6. Oven Drying:

Oven drying is another option for quickly drying herbs. Spread herbs in a single layer on a baking sheet and place them in the oven at a low temperature (around 180°F or 80°C). Keep the oven door slightly ajar to allow moisture to escape. Check frequently to prevent overheating.

7. Testing Dryness:

Regardless of the drying method used, it's crucial to ensure herbs are completely dry before storage. Test for dryness by crumbling a leaf or flower between your fingers. If the herb crumbles easily, it is dry and ready for storage. If it feels moist or leathery, further drying is required.

8. Storage Containers:

Selecting the right storage containers is essential for preserving the quality of dried herbs. Use airtight glass jars or containers to prevent moisture and air from degrading the herbs over time. Avoid plastic containers, as they may not provide an effective barrier against moisture and can leach chemicals into the herbs.

9. Dark and Cool Storage:

Store dried herbs in a cool, dark place away from direct sunlight. Exposure to light can degrade the herbs' essential oils and reduce their potency. A pantry, cupboard, or drawer is an ideal location for storing dried herbs. Maintain a consistent temperature to prevent fluctuations that could impact herb quality.

10. Labeling:

Properly labeling stored herbs is crucial for easy identification. Include the herb's name and the date of harvest on each container. This information helps you track freshness and ensures you use herbs within their optimal period.

11. Whole or Crushed Leaves:

Choose between storing whole leaves or crushing them before storage, depending on your preferences and intended uses. While whole leaves may retain their essential oils better, crushed leaves release flavors more quickly when used in culinary applications or herbal infusions. Adjust the preparation based on your individual preferences.

12. Avoiding Cross-Contamination:

To prevent cross-contamination of flavors, store different herbs in separate containers. Strongly scented herbs, such as mint or rosemary, can impart their aromas to more delicately flavored herbs if stored together. Keep each herb in its dedicated container to preserve its unique characteristics.

13. Check for Mold or Moisture:

Regularly inspect stored herbs for any signs of mold, moisture, or discoloration. If you notice any issues, discard the affected herbs to prevent contamination of the entire storage batch. Maintaining a dry environment and using proper storage containers minimizes the risk of mold growth.

14. Avoiding Crushing:

Handle dried herbs with care to avoid unnecessary crushing. Crushing herbs before use releases their essential oils, and doing so prematurely can lead to flavor and aroma loss. Crush or grind herbs just before use to maximize their freshness and potency.

15. Periodic Rotation and Use:

Herbs, like any other consumable item, have a shelf life. Periodically rotate stored herbs to ensure you use older batches first. This practice helps maintain a fresh supply of herbs and prevents the accumulation of unused, potentially stale products.

Making Herbal Teas and Infusions

Herbal teas and infusions have been cherished for centuries, not just for their delightful flavors but also for their medicinal properties. Steeping a variety of herbs in hot water creates a symphony of tastes and aromas, offering a soothing and healthful experience. In this exploration of making herbal teas and infusions, we delve into the art of blending, brewing, and reaping the numerous benefits these concoctions offer.

Understanding Herbal Teas and Infusions:

Herbal teas and infusions are often used interchangeably, yet they differ in their preparation and purpose. Herbal teas typically involve steeping leaves, flowers, or other plant parts in hot water, creating a delightful beverage. On the other hand, infusions involve a longer steeping time and often include more substantial plant parts like roots or bark, extracting a richer concentration of flavors and beneficial compounds.

Choosing the Right Herbs:

The key to crafting a delightful herbal tea or infusion lies in selecting the right herbs. Beginners may find comfort in familiar herbs like chamomile, peppermint, or lavender. Each herb carries its unique set of properties, from calming chamomile to invigorating peppermint. Experimenting with different combinations allows you to tailor your brew to your taste preferences and health needs.

Herbal Tea Blends:

Creating herbal tea blends is an art that lets you tailor your beverage to your liking. Consider combining herbs with complementary flavors and benefits. A popular calming blend might include chamomile, lavender, and lemon balm. For an energizing morning brew, try mixing peppermint, rosemary, and a touch of citrus zest. The possibilities are endless, and experimenting with various combinations is part of the joy of crafting herbal teas.

Proper Brewing Techniques:

Brewing herbal teas and infusions involves a delicate dance of time and temperature. Boiling water may be suitable for robust herbs like rosemary or thyme, but more delicate varieties such as chamomile or hibiscus require gentler treatment. Generally, a temperature just below boiling is recommended for most herbal concoctions. Steeping times vary, with some teas requiring only a few minutes while infusions may need a more extended period to extract their full essence.

Unleashing Medicinal Properties:

Beyond their exquisite taste, herbal teas and infusions are celebrated for their medicinal properties. Chamomile, known for its calming effect, aids in relaxation and sleep. Peppermint can soothe digestive discomfort, while ginger offers warmth and helps alleviate nausea. Harnessing these natural remedies in the form of a comforting beverage makes incorporating medicinal herbs into your daily routine a delightful experience.

Crafting a Ritual:

Making herbal teas and infusions is not just about brewing a beverage; it's a ritual that engages the senses. The gentle rustle of herbs being measured, the enticing aroma as hot water meets leaves, and the meditative act of sipping a warm cup – all contribute to a mindful experience. Whether it's a morning pick-me-up or an evening wind-down, the ritual of preparing and savoring herbal teas can be a soothing anchor in our fast-paced lives.

The world of herbal teas and infusions is a vast and aromatic realm waiting to be explored. From the selection of herbs to the brewing process, each step offers an opportunity to craft a beverage that not only tantalizes the taste buds but also nurtures the body and soul. As you embark on your journey of herbal concoctions, embrace the creativity, experiment with flavors, and savor the delightful symphony of nature's remedies in a cup.

Choosing Herbs for Tea Blends

In the world of herbal tea blends, the choice of herbs is akin to selecting notes for a melody. Each herb contributes its unique flavor profile, aroma, and potential health benefits, culminating in a harmonious brew that delights the senses. Understanding the characteristics of individual herbs and how they complement each other is key to crafting a tea blend that is both satisfying and purposeful.

Understanding Individual Herbs:

Before delving into the art of blending, it's essential to familiarize oneself with the distinct qualities of various herbs.

Some herbs, like chamomile, impart a subtle floral sweetness, while others, such as peppermint, bring invigorating coolness. Herbal selections like lavender can introduce a soothing, aromatic note, while citrusy herbs like lemongrass add a zesty brightness. Each herb contributes not only to the taste but also to the overall experience of the tea.

Complementary Flavor Profiles:

Creating a well-balanced herbal tea blend is about finding herbs with complementary flavor profiles. For instance, the earthy undertones of rooibos might pair wonderfully with the citrusy notes of orange peel. The warmth of cinnamon can be balanced by the crispness of mint. As you experiment, consider the interplay of sweet, bitter, floral, and spicy elements to achieve a blend that appeals to your palate.

Considering Health Benefits:

Beyond taste, the medicinal properties of herbs add depth and purpose to tea blends. Some herbs are renowned for their calming effects, making them ideal for evening blends or relaxation teas. Others, like ginger and turmeric, bring anti-inflammatory properties, contributing to wellness-focused concoctions. Understanding the health benefits of each herb allows you to tailor your blends to address specific needs or simply enhance overall well-being.

Experimenting with Ratios:

The beauty of crafting herbal tea blends lies in the freedom to experiment with ratios. Start with a base herb that forms the foundation of your blend, considering its dominant flavor and characteristics. Then, add complementary herbs in varying proportions, adjusting to achieve the desired balance. Keep notes on your experiments, as this will guide you in refining your blends over time.

Seasonal Considerations:

The availability and freshness of herbs can vary with the seasons, offering an opportunity to create seasonal tea blends. In the spring, you might explore blends with floral notes from freshly bloomed herbs, while autumn invites the richness of spices like cinnamon and cloves. Embracing the seasonal bounty not only ensures the freshness of your ingredients but also connects you with the rhythms of nature.

Cultural Inspirations:

Drawing inspiration from different cultures can add a fascinating dimension to your herbal tea blends. Explore traditional combinations from around the world, such as the Moroccan blend of mint and green tea or the Ayurvedic blend of holy basil, cardamom, and ginger. Infusing your blends with a cultural touch can transport you to different corners of the globe with each sip.

Choosing herbs for tea blends is an art that involves a thoughtful combination of flavors, aromas, and health benefits. As you embark on this journey of sensory exploration, allow your creativity to flourish, and don't be afraid to push the boundaries of conventional pairings. Whether you're crafting a calming bedtime blend or an invigorating morning elixir, the world of herbal teas invites you to savor the diversity of nature in every cup.

Proper Brewing Techniques

Brewing herbal teas is a delicate dance between science and art, where the proper technique transforms a handful of dried leaves into a fragrant elixir. The right combination of water temperature, steeping time, and method can unlock the full spectrum of flavors and medicinal properties within each herb. In this exploration of proper brewing techniques, we delve into the alchemy that turns herbs into a sensory delight.

The Importance of Water Temperature:

The foundation of a well-brewed herbal tea lies in the choice of water temperature. Different herbs require different temperatures to release their optimal flavors and beneficial compounds. Boiling water is suitable for heartier herbs like rosemary or thyme, while more delicate varieties such as chamomile or green tea prefer water just below boiling to preserve their subtle nuances. Understanding the temperature preferences of your chosen herbs is the first step towards a successful brew.

Mindful Steeping Times:

Steeping time is a critical factor that can make the difference between a perfectly infused tea and a bitter, overpowering concoction. Herbal teas generally require shorter steeping times compared to traditional teas. While some robust herbs, like peppermint, may only need a few minutes, others, such as lavender or chamomile, benefit from a slightly longer infusion. Oversteeping can lead to a bitter taste, so finding the right balance ensures a harmonious blend of flavors.

Choosing the Right Infuser or Strainer:

The vessel in which herbs are steeped plays a vital role in the brewing process. Whether using a traditional teapot, an infuser ball, or a simple strainer, the goal is to allow the herbs ample room to expand and infuse the water. Avoid overcrowding the herbs, as this can result in uneven brewing and a less flavorful tea. Experiment with different infusers to find the one that suits your preferred brewing method and herb choices.

Exploring Cold Infusions:

While hot brewing is the traditional method, cold infusions offer a refreshing alternative, especially in warmer months. Cold brewing involves steeping herbs in cold water for an extended period, typically overnight. This gentle process extracts flavors without the risk of bitterness. Cold-infused herbal teas can be a delightful way to enjoy the subtle notes of herbs like hibiscus, mint, or fruit-infused blends.

Multiple Infusions:

Certain herbs have the ability to yield multiple infusions, allowing you to extract the full potential from your tea leaves. Herbs like oolong or jasmine can be steeped multiple times, each infusion revealing a different facet of their flavor profile. Experiment with extending the brewing time or adjusting the water temperature for subsequent infusions to explore the depth and complexity of your chosen herbs.

Ceremony and Mindfulness:

Brewing herbal tea is not merely a task but a ritual that invites mindfulness. Take a moment to appreciate the aroma of the dry herbs, the gradual unfurling of leaves, and the infusion of color as hot water meets herbs. Engage your senses in the process, and let the act of brewing become a moment of relaxation and reflection.

Proper brewing techniques elevate the simple act of making tea into an art form. By understanding the nuances of water temperature, steeping times, and infusion methods, you can transform a handful of herbs into a symphony of flavors that dance on your palate. Embrace the ritual of brewing, experiment with different techniques, and let the alchemy of herbal teas unfold in each cup.

Creating Homemade Salves and Tinctures

In herbal wellness, the art of creating homemade salves and tinctures is a deeply satisfying endeavor. Beyond the convenience of store-bought remedies, making your own herbal preparations allows you to harness the healing power of plants in a personalized and sustainable way. In this exploration, we delve into the alchemical process of crafting salves and tinctures, transforming herbs into potent balms for body and soul.

Understanding Salves and Tinctures:

Before delving into the crafting process, it's crucial to understand the distinction between salves and tinctures. Salves are topical ointments typically made by infusing herbs into oils and then blending them with beeswax to create a semi-solid, soothing balm. Tinctures, on the other hand, are liquid extracts of herbs, usually preserved in alcohol or glycerin. While tinctures are ingested for their medicinal benefits, salves are applied externally to the skin, offering targeted relief.

Choosing the Right Herbs:

The key to crafting effective salves and tinctures lies in selecting the right herbs. Consider the specific properties of each herb and how they align with your wellness goals. Calendula is renowned for its skin-healing properties, while arnica is favored for its anti-inflammatory effects. Experiment with combinations of herbs to create synergy, enhancing the overall efficacy of your homemade remedies.

Infusing Oils for Salves:

To create a salve, the first step involves infusing herbs into a carrier oil. Choose a high-quality oil such as olive, coconut, or jojoba, known for their skin-nourishing properties. Dried herbs are typically used for infusions to minimize water content, reducing the risk of spoilage. Allow the herbs to steep in the oil over a low heat source or using the solar infusion method, letting the sun gently extract their beneficial compounds.

The Beeswax Connection:

Once the herbal infusion has reached its peak potency, it's time to transform the oil into a salve by adding beeswax. Beeswax provides the desired consistency, turning the infused oil into a spreadable balm. The amount of beeswax used determines the solidity of the salve, allowing you to tailor the texture to your preference. The resulting concoction is not only therapeutic but also a fragrant and tactile pleasure to apply.

Mastering Tincture Extraction:

Creating tinctures involves extracting the medicinal compounds from herbs using alcohol or glycerin as a solvent. High-proof alcohol, such as vodka or brandy, is a popular choice due to its ability to effectively extract a wide range of plant constituents. Finely chop or grind the herbs to increase surface area, facilitating a more efficient extraction. Allow the mixture to macerate for several weeks, shaking it periodically to encourage thorough extraction.

Straining and Bottling:

Once the infusions for both salves and tinctures are complete, the next step is to strain the mixture to remove the plant material. For salves, this means separating the infused oil from the herbs, while tinctures involve filtering out the liquid from the herb-alcohol or herb-glycerin blend. The strained liquid is then bottled, ready for use.

Customizing Your Remedies:

The beauty of crafting homemade salves and tinctures lies in the ability to tailor them to your specific needs. Experiment with different herb combinations, adjusting ratios based on personal preferences and intended uses. Adding essential oils to your salves not only enhances the aroma but also contributes additional therapeutic properties. Consider your skin type, wellness goals, and scent preferences when customizing your herbal creations.

Embracing Sustainable Wellness:

Beyond the therapeutic benefits, crafting homemade remedies embodies a sustainable approach to wellness. Growing your own herbs or sourcing them from reputable sources allows you to connect with the earth and reduce reliance on commercially produced products. This conscious, hands-on approach to herbalism fosters a deeper understanding of the plants and their healing potential.

Creating homemade salves and tinctures is a journey into the heart of herbal alchemy. From selecting the right herbs to infusing oils and crafting personalized remedies, the process is a celebration of the healing gifts nature provides.

Whether you seek relief for aching muscles, skincare solutions, or overall well-being, the art of crafting salves and tinctures invites you to explore the richness of herbal remedies from the comfort of your kitchen.

Medicinal Properties of Different Herbs

Herbs have been cherished for centuries not only for their culinary appeal but also for their potent medicinal properties. From soothing teas to healing salves, the diverse world of herbs offers a natural pharmacy for various ailments. In this exploration, we delve into the rich tapestry of medicinal properties found in different herbs, uncovering the age-old wisdom that continues to resonate in modern herbalism.

1. Chamomile (Matricaria chamomilla):

Calming and Anti-inflammatory: Chamomile is renowned for its calming properties, making it a popular choice for promoting relaxation and alleviating stress. Its anti-inflammatory and anti-spasmodic effects also extend to aiding digestion and relieving gastrointestinal discomfort.

2. Peppermint (Mentha x piperita):

Digestive Aid and Energizing: Peppermint is a versatile herb known for its refreshing flavor and numerous health benefits. It helps soothe digestive issues, alleviate nausea, and relieve headaches. Additionally, peppermint has energizing properties, making it an excellent choice for a revitalizing herbal infusion.

3. Lavender (Lavandula angustifolia):

Calming and Antiseptic: Lavender's aromatic blooms are not only pleasing to the senses but also possess calming properties. It is commonly used in aromatherapy to promote relaxation and improve sleep quality. Topically, lavender exhibits antiseptic and anti-inflammatory qualities, making it a valuable addition to salves and balms.

4. Echinacea (Echinacea purpurea):

Immune-Boosting: Echinacea is celebrated for its immune-boosting properties. It stimulates the production of white blood cells and enhances the body's ability to fend off infections. This herb is often used to reduce the severity and duration of colds and flu.

5. Turmeric (Curcuma longa):

Anti-inflammatory and Antioxidant: The vibrant golden spice, turmeric, contains curcumin, a compound with potent anti-inflammatory and antioxidant properties. It is widely used to alleviate joint pain, reduce inflammation, and support overall immune health.

6. Ginger (Zingiber officinale):

Anti-nausea and Anti-inflammatory: Ginger is renowned for its digestive benefits, particularly in alleviating nausea and indigestion. It also exhibits anti-inflammatory properties, making it a natural remedy for conditions such as arthritis and muscle soreness.

7. Rosemary (Rosmarinus officinalis):

Memory and Circulation Support: Beyond its culinary uses, rosemary has been traditionally associated with memory enhancement. It is believed to improve concentration and support overall cognitive function. Rosemary also has circulation-boosting properties, aiding in cardiovascular health.

8. Holy Basil (Ocimum sanctum):

Adaptogenic and Stress-Relieving: Holy Basil, also known as Tulsi, is revered for its adaptogenic properties, helping the body adapt to stress and maintain balance. It is commonly used to alleviate anxiety, support the immune system, and promote overall well-being.

9. Valerian (Valeriana officinalis):

Relaxant and Sleep Aid: Valerian is a well-known herb for its calming and sedative effects. It is often used as a natural remedy for insomnia and anxiety, promoting relaxation and improving sleep quality.

10. Arnica (Arnica montana):

Anti-inflammatory and Pain Relief: Arnica is a popular herb for external use, especially in the form of creams or ointments. It is known for its anti-inflammatory properties and is commonly used topically to relieve pain and swelling associated with bruises, sprains, and muscle soreness.

The medicinal properties of herbs are a testament to the profound healing potential found in nature. Each herb brings a unique set of benefits, and the art of herbalism involves understanding their properties and synergies. Whether sipped as a tea, applied topically, or incorporated into culinary creations, the diverse world of herbs offers a holistic approach to health and well-being.

As with any form of natural medicine, it's advisable to consult with a healthcare professional before incorporating herbs into your wellness routine, especially if you have underlying health conditions or are taking medications.

Step-by-Step Instructions

Step-by-step instructions are the unsung heroes of our daily lives, guiding us through a myriad of tasks, from assembling furniture to mastering a new recipe. They provide a structured pathway, demystifying complex processes and empowering individuals to accomplish goals with confidence. In this exploration, we dive into the art of crafting effective step-by-step instructions, understanding their importance, and unraveling the nuances that elevate them from mere directions to empowering guides.

1. Clarity is Key:

Begin with a clear and concise introduction that outlines the goal or objective of the task at hand. Clearly state what the reader will achieve by following the instructions. Ambiguity can lead to confusion, so ensure that your language is straightforward and easily comprehensible. A well-defined objective sets the tone for the entire set of instructions.

2. Break it Down:

Divide the task into manageable steps. Each step should represent a specific action or subtask that contributes to the overall completion of the goal. Breaking down the process into smaller, digestible parts makes it easier for the reader to follow and reduces the likelihood of feeling overwhelmed.

3. Provide Visual Aids:

A picture is worth a thousand words. Whenever possible, incorporate visual aids such as diagrams, illustrations, or photographs. Visual representations enhance clarity and serve as a valuable supplement to the written instructions. Visual aids are particularly beneficial for tasks that involve physical manipulation or spatial orientation.

4. Sequential Flow:

Maintain a logical sequence throughout the instructions. Ensure that the steps follow a chronological order that mirrors the natural progression of the task. This sequential flow assists readers in understanding the dependencies between steps and helps them anticipate what comes next.

5. Anticipate Challenges:

Consider potential challenges or questions that may arise during the execution of each step. Address these concerns preemptively within the instructions. Providing troubleshooting tips or clarifications demonstrates foresight and ensures that users can navigate through potential obstacles with confidence.

6. Use Consistent Language:

Maintain consistency in your choice of language and terminology. This applies not only to the step-by-step instructions but also to any labels, captions, or terminology used throughout the document. Consistency fosters clarity and prevents confusion arising from conflicting terminology.

7. Incorporate Action Verbs:

Use action verbs to convey the intended actions clearly. Action verbs provide a sense of direction and leave no room for ambiguity. Instead of passive language, opt for active phrasing that empowers the reader to take decisive steps. For example, "Insert the tab into the slot" is more direct than "The tab should be inserted into the slot."

8. Test and Iterate:

Before finalizing your step-by-step instructions, conduct a trial run of the task yourself or have someone else follow the instructions. This practical testing phase allows you to identify any ambiguities, omissions, or areas that may need clarification. Use feedback to refine and iterate the instructions for optimal clarity.

9. Encourage Confidence:

Throughout the instructions, foster a sense of confidence and reassurance. Use positive language that motivates the reader, and offer encouragement along the way. A confident reader is more likely to successfully complete the task, and positive reinforcement contributes to a positive user experience.

10. Conclusion and Next Steps:

Conclude the set of instructions with a summary or recap of the completed task. Reinforce the accomplishment of the goal and express confidence in the reader's abilities. If applicable, provide information on what to do next or any additional steps to enhance the user's experience.

In a world often characterized by the hustle and bustle of modern living, the allure of medicinal herbs beckons, offering a natural and holistic approach to well-being. Beyond their traditional use in teas and remedies, medicinal herbs can seamlessly integrate into everyday life, enhancing both health and culinary experiences. In this exploration, we uncover the art of incorporating medicinal herbs into daily routines, transforming ordinary moments into opportunities for nourishment and healing.

1. Morning Rituals with Herbal Teas:

Start your day on a soothing note by incorporating herbal teas into your morning routine. Choose herbs such as peppermint or ginger for an invigorating wake-up call or opt for calming chamomile to ease into the day. A warm cup of herbal tea not only hydrates but also introduces medicinal properties that set a positive tone for the day.

2. Culinary Adventures with Fresh Herbs:

Elevate your culinary creations by infusing them with the vibrant flavors of fresh herbs. Basil, rosemary, thyme, and cilantro not only add depth and aroma to dishes but also bring their unique medicinal benefits. Create herb-infused oils, toss fresh leaves into salads, or use them as garnishes to unleash the herbal symphony on your taste buds.

3. Herbal Tonics for Hydration:

Ditch the sugary beverages and opt for herbal tonics to stay hydrated throughout the day. Infuse water with slices of cucumber, mint, and a hint of lemon for a refreshing and healthful alternative. This simple herbal infusion not only quenches thirst but also provides a subtle boost of vitamins and antioxidants.

4. Relaxation with Herbal Baths:

Transform your evening bath into a therapeutic ritual by adding a blend of medicinal herbs. Lavender, chamomile, and calendula petals create a soothing and aromatic concoction that promotes relaxation. The herbal infusion not only nurtures the skin but also calms the mind, making it an ideal way to unwind after a busy day.

5. Herbal Infused Honey:

Upgrade your sweeteners by infusing honey with medicinal herbs. Choose herbs like thyme or lavender and let them steep in honey for a few weeks. The result is a delicately flavored herbal honey that can be drizzled over desserts, added to tea, or enjoyed on its own for a delightful burst of natural sweetness with added health benefits.

6. Aromatherapy with Herbal Sachets:

Introduce the calming scents of medicinal herbs into your living spaces with herbal sachets. Create sachets using dried herbs like rosemary, lavender, or eucalyptus, and place them in drawers, closets, or under pillows. The gentle aroma not only freshens up your surroundings but also contributes to a serene and stress-free atmosphere.

7. Herbal Skincare Rituals:

Nourish your skin with the healing properties of herbs by incorporating them into your skincare routine. Calendula and chamomile are known for their soothing effects, making them excellent additions to homemade creams or face masks. Harnessing the power of herbs in skincare enhances natural radiance and promotes overall skin health.

8. Herbal Energizers for Afternoon Slumps:

Combat the mid-afternoon energy slump with herbal energizers. Create a blend of herbs like ginseng, rosemary, and peppermint for a revitalizing infusion. This herbal pick-me-up provides a natural and sustained energy boost without the jitters associated with caffeine, making it a healthier alternative to afternoon coffees.

9. Mindful Meditation with Herbal Scents:

Engage in mindful meditation with the aid of herbal scents. Essential oils from herbs like lavender, frankincense, or sage can be diffused during meditation sessions, creating a serene ambiance and enhancing the overall experience. The aromatic embrace of medicinal herbs contributes to mental clarity and relaxation.

10. Herb-Infused Sleep Rituals:

Wrap up your day with a soothing sleep ritual infused with herbs known for their calming properties. A cup of chamomile tea, a lavender-infused pillow mist, or a few drops of valerian tincture can promote restful sleep. Integrating herbal elements into your nighttime routine transforms the act of winding down into a gentle and nourishing experience.

Beauty and Health Products

In a world filled with commercial beauty and health products laden with synthetic ingredients, the allure of do-it-yourself (DIY) formulations beckons. Harnessing the potency of natural ingredients, DIY beauty and health products allow individuals to create personalized and nourishing concoctions that cater to their unique needs. In this exploration, we unveil the art of crafting DIY beauty and health products, unlocking the transformative potential of nature's bounty.

1. The Allure of Homemade Skincare:

Embarking on a DIY skincare journey opens the door to a realm of possibilities. Create a rejuvenating face mask with ingredients like honey, yogurt, and turmeric for a radiant glow. Formulate a gentle exfoliator using sugar, coconut oil, and a dash of essential oils. The simplicity of homemade skincare products allows for tailored solutions that cater to individual skin types and concerns.

2. Natural Hair Care Elixirs:

Bid farewell to commercial hair products laden with chemicals and embrace the natural goodness of DIY hair care elixirs. Formulate a nourishing hair mask using ingredients like avocado, coconut oil, and honey to replenish moisture and restore luster. Create a herbal-infused hair rinse with chamomile or rosemary for added shine and scalp health. DIY hair care empowers individuals to tailor formulations based on hair type, texture, and specific needs.

3. Soothing Herbal Salves and Balms:

Healing and nourishing, DIY herbal salves and balms are crafted to address a variety of skin concerns. Calendula-infused salves can soothe irritated skin, while lavender and chamomile balms offer relaxation and relief. The process of creating these balms fosters a deeper connection with the healing properties of herbs, transforming skincare routines into moments of self-care.

4. Holistic Oral Care Products:

Extend the DIY ethos to oral care with natural and holistic alternatives. Create a simple toothpaste using baking soda, coconut oil, and peppermint essential oil. Formulate mouthwash with antiseptic herbs like sage and thyme for a refreshing and germ-fighting solution. DIY oral care products not only contribute to a healthier mouth but also reduce exposure to potentially harmful additives found in commercial alternatives.

5. Therapeutic Bath Bombs and Salts:

Elevate bath time into a therapeutic ritual by crafting DIY bath bombs and salts. Blend Epsom salt with essential oils like lavender or eucalyptus for a soothing soak that relaxes muscles and relieves stress. Personalizing scents and ingredients allows for a sensorial escape, transforming the bathroom into a spa-like sanctuary.

6. Essential Oil Blends for Well-Being:

Delve into the world of aromatherapy by creating personalized essential oil blends. Blend calming lavender and bergamot for a stress-relieving rollerball, or combine invigorating peppermint and citrus oils for an energizing diffuser blend. DIY essential oil creations offer a fragrant and natural way to support emotional well-being and enhance mood.

7. Herbal Infusions for Internal Health:

Extend the benefits of DIY to internal health with herbal infusions. Create soothing teas using herbs like chamomile, ginger, or peppermint for digestive wellness. Craft herbal tinctures with ingredients like elderberry or echinacea to support the immune system. DIY herbal infusions provide a gentle yet effective approach to internal health, allowing individuals to tailor blends based on specific health goals.

8. Natural Deodorants and Body Sprays:

Bid farewell to commercial deodorants with potentially harmful ingredients by crafting natural alternatives at home. Mix baking soda, cornstarch, and coconut oil for a simple yet effective DIY deodorant. Create a refreshing body spray with aloe vera, witch hazel, and your favorite essential oils for a personalized fragrance that lingers throughout the day.

9. DIY Sleep Rituals:

Cultivate a restful night's sleep with DIY sleep rituals. Craft a calming pillow mist with lavender and chamomile to promote relaxation. Formulate a bedtime tea blend with herbs like valerian, passionflower, and lemon balm for a tranquil pre-sleep routine. DIY sleep rituals harness the power of herbs to create a serene and supportive environment for restorative sleep.

10. Sustainable Living with DIY Products:

Beyond the immediate benefits to personal well-being, DIY beauty and health products contribute to a more sustainable lifestyle. By utilizing natural and locally sourced ingredients, individuals reduce their environmental footprint and minimize exposure to potentially harmful chemicals found in conventional products. This eco-conscious approach aligns with the principles of mindful living and fosters a deeper connection with nature.